ELECTRO ACUPUNCTURE BY VOLL (EAV) AND HOMEOPATHY

By Nadejda G. Grigorova, Ph.D.

ELECTRO ACUPUNCTURE BY VOLL (EAV) AND HOMEOPATHY

By Nadejda G. Grigorova, Ph.D.

All identifying details, including names have been changed to protect patient confidentiality.

The information in this book does not contradict the diagnosis and treatment methods of modern allopathic medicine. This book is not intended as a substitute for advice from a trained professional. The author and the publisher are not responsible for cases of self-diagnosis and self-treatment. They recommend consultation with a medical or a naturopathic doctor in every case of a health problem.

ISBN 978-0-9854390-0-2
Library of Congress Control Number: 2012906458

Published in the United States of America
by Milkana Publishing, Santa Clara, California
First Edition in English

Originally published in Bulgarian by Shambala Books, Ltd.,
Sofia, Bulgaria, 2007

TABLE OF CONTENTS

ACKNOWLEDGMENTS

Throughout my life and while writing this book, I have had many experiences and met many people for whom I am grateful. My grandmother, Neda Prodanova, taught me that there is real healing power in Nature, and for this I owe her a debt of gratitude. I am grateful to my family and to my children, Milkana and Ivan, for their trust in me and the path that I followed in my life.

I am grateful to Peter Chappel who came to Bulgaria from London as a real apostle, inspiring many people to learn about homeopathy and who opened new horizons for us. He changed my life.

I must not forget to thank Mrs. Angela Needham, who came from England during the most difficult time of change in our country, after the fall of the Berlin Wall when Sofia was short of water, electricity, and bread. During this tumultuous time, she was our teacher in the practice of homeopathy. Many thanks are due to my teacher in Voll testing, Alexander Vlahov, who keeps in touch and continues to introduce me to the latest achievements of this method in Russia. I am thankful for his permission to use the description of the measurement points found in his *Principles of Bioresonance Diagnosis* [Tanev & Vlahov, 1995].

Thanks also to Mrs. Chamilla Sanua for her enthusiasm as she continues to search for new natural remedies at Weleda Pharmacies in Johannesburg. She converted Weleda into an institution of natural healing. I am very thankful to my clients who have trusted my knowledge and followed my diets and recommendations religiously, even when they were not easy to follow. I send my blessings to the young engineer Ivan Kirilov Grigorov for the small, but very sensitive Bulgarian Voll machine IKG-1, which has given me no problems during fifteen years of heavy use.

For help editing this book I am thankful forever to Mrs. Mohsina Honnorat, a student in homeopathy and my dear friend. I thank Dr. Jean Donaldson for the strict, scientific, yet broadminded criticisms and suggestions and for assisting my attempts to write in English.

For this first edition in the United States of America, I owe many thanks to my daughter, Milkana Grigorova, for taking this book through all stages of publishing and to my copyeditor Kathleen Erickson, for her high professionalism, sunny disposition and relentless answering many editorial questions.

I am grateful to my friends from Bulgaria and from South Africa who always supported me and who helped me to believe in myself during some of the hardest times in my life. Thank you to everyone, many times over.

PREFACE

Until I was in my forties I did not know much about homeopathy. In Bulgaria, my country, this method of healing was almost unknown during the time of communism.

My contact with the art of healing was through my grandmother, Neda Prodanova. She lived in a little town, Varbitza, in the eastern part of the Balkan Mountains. For many years she would pick herbs and use them to heal people. As a child, I spent every summer holiday with her from June to September. This was my favorite time of year, with flowers and sunny meadows, and the smell of herbs everywhere. My grandmother showed me different plants and explained their properties. My interest in herbs was strong. I read my grandmother's books, and later as a student in chemistry at the University of Sofia I bought many books on phytotherapy. Later, I worked for twenty five years in the Bulgarian Academy of Science as a research fellow in the analytical chemistry of metals. I never thought that I would eventually end up working in the field of natural medicine.

At the end of April 1986, the explosion of the nuclear power station in Chernobyl, in the Ukraine, resulted in a real disaster for Europe. A radioactive cloud covered most of the continent.

At that time, the communist government of Bulgaria kept this terrible event a secret for three days, and emergency measures were not implemented efficiently. It happened during a long holiday and I worked outdoors in my garden. I was not aware that the constant drizzle of rain that day, May 1, 1986, was polluted with radioactivity. During the next few days, the signal for radioactivity from the Geiger counter in our laboratory was so loud that we simply switched it off.

Like many other people in my country, I was badly affected by the dose of radiation. A month later I had no energy and a blood test showed I had reached a dangerous level of leukopenia. I began treatment with medication immediately and continued for more than a year. During that long year, I was sure that things were not going well for me because every time I stopped the treatment, the leukocyte count dropped again. I started thinking seriously about my life and possible death. There were many things I had

11

wanted to do that I had not yet done. Other things that I previously thought were important, I realized really didn't matter.

I began to prioritize and I realized with certainty that I wanted to build a house in the mountains near Sofia and that I also wanted to finish the thesis for my Ph.D. degree. I hid my real condition from my family, and I continued working in the laboratory, working on my dissertation, and organizing the building of a new house in the mountains. These activities needed so much energy and attention that I had no time to think about death at all. The following year my health improved greatly.

I succeeded in building a house and obtained a Ph.D. degree, but I was not the same person. My thinking was different. My outlook on life and my values had changed.

In trying to improve my health, I read most of the University's medical books. As a scientist I was not satisfied with the scientific level of these books. The paradigm of conventional medicine was based on the Newtonian physical model, very different from the achievements of quantum physics and contemporary chemistry.

Step by step during the next few years, I attended courses in traditional Chinese medicine and acupuncture, bioenergetics, and herbalism, and eventually attended a course in homeopathy.

At that time in 1993, the London College of Classical Homeopathy (LCCH) undertook a mission to the East European countries, including Bulgaria.

The young Bulgarian medical doctors Dr. Petar Naidenov, Dr. Dora Patchova, and Dr. Atanas Galabov, members of the Center for Natural Healing "Anhira," invited Mr. Peter Chappel, Director of the London College of Classical Homeopathy (LCCH), to lecture in homeopathy in my home city of Sofia. By pure chance I attended that lecture.

That chance meeting opened the door for a regular two-year course in homeopathy, followed by another two years of lectures in general medicine following the curriculum of the LCCH. In this way, I graduated from the London College of Classical Homeopathy with the first homeopaths to complete the course in Bulgaria. The LCCH continued its mission to Bulgaria until three course cycles had been given.

Three months before our graduation, together with Dr. Violeta Djerekarova, we published a student manual, *Introduction to Homeopathic Materia Medica,* for the next Bulgarian students to use in the subsequent

12

courses on homeopathy. This book was an expression of my enthusiasm for the subject matter found in *Homeopathic Materia Medica*, which is a collection of knowledge about homeopathic remedies along with wisdom about human nature.

I continued working at the Bulgarian Academy of Science during the day. In the evenings I practiced homeopathy at a private clinic, Gracia, directed by Professor Dr. Topuzov, in Sofia. I was delighted to do this work, and I examined the results very critically. I saw numerous miraculous healings with homeopathic remedies, and this convinced me that homeopathic remedies could work.

Thinking about every step of the homeopathic treatment, I realized that the method for choosing a remedy was not precise. The "prescription" depended on the practitioner and was an expression of his knowledge, preferences, prejudice, and opinion. The lack of process could result in a choice of remedy that was not the simillimum (the best one).

For this reason, in 1996 I attended a course in Bio-Resonance Medicine and Electro-Acupuncture by Voll (EAV), organized by the Bulgarian Homeopathic Society in Sofia. The lecturer was Mr. Alexander Vlahov, a follower of the Russian school in Voll testing. The course provided an opportunity to develop a new method for choosing a homeopathic remedy; we learned to test the remedy's particular action on a specific individual. For some time after that course, I continued practicing homeopathy in the old classical way involving a homeopathic interview. However, from time to time I used the Voll machine to test the major organs of the patient and to check their condition.

In 1997, I immigrated to the Republic of South Africa. Homeopathy is recognized as a viable medical option in South Africa, where many people prefer to take natural and homeopathic remedies. Weleda Pharmacies has an excellent reputation and is well-known as a good source of medicine and advice. Soon after I arrived, I found a job with a Weleda Pharmacy in Bryanston, Johannesburg.

My international diploma in Classical Homeopathy from LCCH was not recognized by the authorities in the Republic of South Africa (RSA), so I could not be registered as a homeopath. (I was accepted later and registered as a natural health practitioner in the RSA.) Voll testing was something new to the country, and it was not included in the regulations of the Allied Health Professions Council of South Africa. But the owner of Weleda

13

Pharmacy, Mrs. Camilla Sanua, believed in me and gave me an opportunity to start allergy testing with the Voll machine. I worked for five years with Mrs. Sanua at Weleda. During that time, I never carried out homeopathic interviews with the clients, but instead tested their organs for imbalances. In the thousands of clients I worked with at Weleda, I observed that the imbalances in specific organs and the presence of different pathogens could cause allergic reactions. While testing homeopathic remedies for balancing the organs and systems, I found that certain remedies had a specific action against certain microorganisms. If a reaction was confirmed for more than five individuals, I put this fact in my notes. Later I realized that these notes were part of a research program.

For a real research project to be completed successfully, it is essential that the work be carried out by a group of practitioners and that the results be statistically evaluated. For this reason I am documenting the pilot research I have already completed in the form of this book. I hope that it will be useful to Voll practitioners for their daily work. I believe that enthusiastic Voll practitioners and Homeopaths will find something interesting in this book and hope some of them will use this information as a basis to continue the research.

I firmly believe that Energy medicine is the future of medicine.

We are made of light. The presence of energy is the most important attribute of life. To restore the health of a body means to restore its energy.

I am positive about the future of medicine. I believe that medicine will become absolutely gentle, noninvasive, and natural.

Nadia Grigorova, Ph.D., May, 2007
Johannesburg, Republic of South Africa
neda46@hotmail.com

PREFACE TO THE 2012 EDITION

In 2008, I returned to Bulgaria from South Africa. I registered as a naturopathic practitioner and, as part of this qualification, I obtained a Bachelor of Science in Pharmacy, from the Medical Academy in Sofia, Bulgaria.

During this time I prepared the first group of Bulgarian students in Voll testing. I would be happy to teach anyone who would like to apply Voll testing in Medicine and Homeopathy. I believe that using Voll testing as a support for Homeopathic practice helps the development of Homeopathic Medicine in the clinical direction; and that it also helps both the Homeopathic and official Allopathic Medicine to come closer together in terms of their understanding of the etiology and the gentle cure of ailments for the benefit of the patients.

> Nadia Grigorova, Ph.D.
> April 2012, Sofia, Bulgaria
> neda46@hotmail.com

INTRODUCTION

Originally this book was printed as a booklet for the Voll testing courses I taught in Johannesburg from 2000 to 2003. In 2004, the text was enlarged and I added many patients' results in the form of case studies.

The first chapter, **WORLD OF ENERGY,** is a short presentation of contemporary cosmic ideas in science. In the 20th century, the Newtonian mechanical model of the world was replaced by relativistic quantum physics. The new model included unity of matter, energy and information, interconnection of the events in our Universe, and the idea that consciousness is an expression of high-vibration energies of an invisible reality. These are the three keys to understanding that every living cell and every organism is a source of signals, which are an integral part of the way a cell functions and communicates with the world.

Traditional Chinese medicine is based on the movement and balance of energies in the human body and corresponds very well to the new cosmic model. However, the Newtonian mechanical model is still the basis of conventional medicine. That paradigm will change, but it will take time.

Chapter Two, **ELECTRO ACUPUNCTURE BY VOLL (EAV),** explains the method of Dr. R. Voll. His method is based on physical measurements of the specific conductivity of the skin in the Chinese meridian points and the new points of the Voll meridians. The discussion includes the process of taking measurements, the required conditions for a good test, normal vs. abnormal readings, and the idea that the readings can be balanced by putting different substances, including homeopathic medicine, in contact with the machine.

The success with patients using EAV indicate that this method could be used successfully in future medical treatments. Based on the teachings of Dr. Voll, the topography of the most commonly used points, 12 Chinese meridians and 8 Voll meridians, is described as well as the relationship of the points and meridians to the organs and systems of the human body.

In the third chapter, **HOMEOPATHY, AN ENERGY MEDICINE**, the leading principles of homeopathy and their relationship with the laws of quantum photochemistry are described. A homeopathic remedy can be considered to be a source of quantum energy. The energy provided can only be absorbed by the organism if it is in resonance with the energy needs of that organism. According to quantum photochemistry, only one quanta of light is necessary and sufficient to induce a molecule to undergo an energy transformation. For this reason, very diluted substances in homeopathy are capable of inducing powerful biochemical transformations in the human organism.

Potentization of a solution, the role of the solvent, and the redistribution of energy within the dissolved molecule are also explained according to quantum photochemistry in the third chapter. The human constitution is considered to be a specific spectrum of vibrating energies, and when deficient these vibrating energies can be supplemented by the proper constitutional remedy. The simillimum is a remedy that can completely supply the energy needs of an individual. One can confirm the spectral reach of a new homeopathic remedy by testing the remedy using healthy volunteers.

The invention of homeopathy and homeopathic remedies is a revolutionary event in medicine. The methods used currently by mainstream homeopathic practitioners are mainly the art of finding the simillimum remedy. Electro Acupuncture by Voll, with its possibility of testing homeopathic remedies, provides a great opportunity for homeopathy to move from its status as an art to that of a modern science.

In the fourth chapter, **THE EAV METHOD AS A SUPPORT FOR HOMEOPATHY**, the principal direction of my research is discussed. It includes: studying the effect of homeopathic remedies on pathogenic microorganisms, confirmed by Voll testing; determination of the spectral frequencies of the activity of some homeopathic remedies by comparison with the known resonant frequencies of pathogens; proving the effectiveness of remedies for treating viral infections; finding homeopathic remedies for balancing the bacterial flora of the gut; the relationship between allergy, pathogenic bowel flora, and disturbances of the functioning of the digestive system; interaction of homeopathic remedies with vitamins, minerals, and other supplements; action of homeopathic nosodes as a source of a specific vibration spectrum; and the use of specific diets during homeopathic treatment.

The results from experimental studies carried out over seven years are shown in five tables in the Appendices. *Table 3* shows **BACTERIAL**

18

AND FUNGAL PATHOGENS AND HOMEOPATHIC REMEDIES CONFIRMED BY EAV TESTS AS SPECIFIC FOR THESE PATHOGENS. The information in this table could be useful to Voll practitioners and to homeopaths as an addition to their repertories (homeopathic reference books). Upgrading the Voll machines' computer programs to add a Custom Library would permit scanning of groups of different pathogens for the proven specific homeopathic remedies.

Table 4 collects information about **BACTERIAL AND FUNGAL PATHOGENS RELATED TO FOOD INTOLERANCE.** This table includes the suggested diets to be followed during treatment.

The results obtained by treatment of viral infections are in *Table 5*: **SOME VIRUSES AND HOMEOPATHIC REMEDIES SPECIFIC FOR THEM AS PROVED BY EAV TESTS.**

At present, diseases caused by a virus are difficult to treat and continue to be a problem for the medical profession. Therefore, the knowledge and use of mild and noninvasive homeopathic remedies for viruses could be helpful for both doctors and alternative healers. Homeopathic remedies work successfully in combination with antioxidants.

Table 6 summarizes the information about the action of some homeopathic remedies used in my practice of Voll testing: **HOMEOPATHIC REMEDIES ACTIVE FOR DIFFERENT PATHOGENS AND THEIR RESONANCE FREQUENCIES.** A method for finding a homeopathic remedy's spectral area of action by using the pathogens' resonance frequencies data found in the literature is described. Some of the results are presented in graphic form and one can see the difference in the spectra of similar remedies belonging to the same group (such as potassium salts or mercury salts).

The results for parasitic infections are presented in *Table 7*: **SOME PARASITES AND HOMEOPATHIC REMEDIES CONFIRMED BY EAV TEST AS SPECIFIC FOR THESE PARASITES.** This table shows the action of homeopathic remedies on parasites such as Amoeba, Ascaris, Toxoplasma, Bilharzia, Trichomonas, and others. The integration of traditional Chinese medicine and homeopathy does not exclude the broad knowledge of conventional medicine.

In the fifth chapter, **EAV AND HOMEOPATHY IN PRACTICE**, pathogens from different families such as Parasites, Bacteria, Viruses, Mycoplasma, Rickettsia, Chlamydia, Mycobacterium, and Fungi are described. The epidemiological and microbiological information is given. The best homeopathic remedies found by Voll tests are listed. Supplements are also mentioned, such as antioxidants, vitamins, and others useful for the treatment of different pathogens. The procedures for allergy testing and detecting imbalances in the organs and systems are described. The pleomorphic theory of Dr. Enderlein is presented as an illustration of the role of the milieu, or the internal environmental conditions, permitting the pathogens to develop.

The last chapter, **CASE STUDIES,** presents 44 real cases of problems solved successfully by using Voll tests in combination with homeopathic and natural remedies.

This book can be used by medical practitioners as a manual for Voll testing. The information can also be used by homeopaths in their clinical practice. And this book can inspire some homeopaths to explore additional new horizons in homeopathy.

CHAPTER 1
WORLD OF ENERGY

1.1. MATTER AND ENERGY

The revolutionary changes in science happen silently. The most brilliant ideas often need the longest time to be accepted. In the beginning of the 20th century with the work of world-famous physicist Albert Einstein, a silent revolution started in the field of science in Europe.

For centuries prior to Einstein the mechanical model of the world as explained by the physical laws of Isaac Newton was accepted. Newton's physical model described the world as a predictable system based on three basic laws:

1) If we know an object's speed and the time of an object's movement in some direction, we can find that object in an exactly predicted place.

2) If force is applied to a particle and its mass is known, we can calculate the acceleration of that particle.

3) For every action, there is an equal and opposite reaction. If an action is applied to an object, an equal reaction appears in the opposite direction.

These physical principles make the world easily understandable. For example, if we apply them to chemistry and to medicine, it sounds like this: "If we give more medicine we get better results." Drug therapy is still a Newtonian model as is the idea of organ transplantation: Replace the broken part of the mechanism. But first in physics, and later in other branches of science, more and more experimental data did not fit the Newtonian model. In 1919 Albert Einstein produced his equation:

$$E = mc^2$$

where: E = energy

m = mass

c = speed of the light in vacuum, 3×10^8 m/s.

This equation expresses that mass is a form of energy. Matter can turn into energy. All matter is accumulated energy. According to Einstein's theory, the speed of light in a vacuum, 3×10^8 m/s, is the upper limit for the speed of any object.

The model of atomic structure developed in the beginning of the 20th century postulated that the atom is like a solar system with a large positive mass in the center and electrons circulating around it. The electrons have a very small mass and a negative charge. The position of the electrons in their orbits is strictly determined and each orbit has its specific energy, which can be released if the electron passes into a lower orbit. At the moment an electron passes into a lower orbit, a portion of energy, a photon (a quantum of light), is released with a very specific frequency. The following equation shows the connection between the energy of the photon and the frequency of the light.

$$E = h \, \nu$$

where: E = energy
h = Planck's constant ($6.62620 . \ 10^{-34}$ J.s)
ν = frequency

The higher the frequency of the light, the higher the energy of the photon.

Scientists have found that a photon has the properties of a particle (it has energy), and at the same time it has the behavior of a wave (it has a specific wavelength and a specific frequency). The wavelength is inversely proportional to its frequency as follows:

$$\lambda = 1 / \nu$$

where: λ = length of the wave
ν = frequency of the wave

Waves are dynamic structures; they oscillate from a low point to the maximum of a sinusoidal curve. Waves interact with each other according to the laws of physics. An interference pattern is the resulting mixed picture when two waves meet and combine in a superimposed fashion. Such a pattern can be seen on the surface of water, for example, when two stones are thrown into the water near each other and the resulting circles meet and overlap.

The resonance frequencies we describe in homeopathy are those frequencies whose vibrations are the same as the vibration spectrum of the receiver (i.e. a person, a machine, a bridge, or any object). For example, if a singer sings in front of a glass, he can cause the glass to break if he produces a note that vibrates at the same frequency as the vibrational resonances of the glass.

The electromagnetic fields created by moving charged particles interact in a similar wave fashion, demonstrating properties of interference and resonance. Energy forms the basis of everything in the world. The energy spectrum has a huge range of frequencies, but our eyes can detect only a limited part of this spectrum corresponding to the perceived colors in order from red, orange, yellow, green, and blue, up to violet. We know other frequencies exist that are invisible to the human eye but detectable by devices: such as radio frequencies, infrared radiation, ultraviolet radiation, X-rays, and gamma rays. Space is full of energy, and some forms of energy are still probably completely unknown to us.

This discussion, when applied to our health and to medicine, shows that if our body works because of energy, then the best way to heal the body is to work to repair and balance the energy of the system.

1.2. THE UNIVERSE IS A GIANT HOLOGRAM

Dr. John Bell (1928–1990) was an Irish physicist who worked in Geneva at CERN, one of the best laboratories in the world for studying the subatomic structure of matter. In 1964 he proved his theorem about nonlocal interaction between subatomic particles.

The nonlocal interaction links up one location with another without crossing space, without decay, and without delay. A nonlocal interaction is immediate, unmitigated, and faster than the speed of light.

Bell's presumption is that quantum physics theory allows for the existence of an invisible reality in which a connection between all material or energy events in the Universe is always present, irrespective of the distance between them. Communication between connected events occurs at a speed faster than the speed of light. Our senses and our physical instruments are not capable of sensing the total amount of vibrations in the Universe. When events communicate instantaneously, we can expect a sequence of cause and effect to happen simultaneously even when they are separated by large distances. For this to be possible everything must be interconnected. This interconnection of everything in time and space

23

is supported by a Holographic model of the world as proposed by some physicists.

At the University of Paris in 1982, the physicist Alain Aspect and his research team discovered that, under certain circumstances, subatomic particles such as electrons are able to communicate with each other regardless of the distance between them and with a speed faster than the speed of light.

This phenomenon is consistent with the theory of a holographic world postulated by David Bohm, a University of London physicist. Bohm believed that the Universe is a gigantic and detailed hologram, where everything interpenetrates everything else [Bohm, 1987]. He theorized that a pilot wave called the quantum potential "Q" emerges from a deeper unobservable domain of the Universe and guides the observed behavior of particles. Later Bohm identified the deeper level of reality as the "implicate order"—a holographic field where all quantum states are permanently coded. Observed reality emerges from this field by a constant unfolding [László, 2004].

Holography is a physical method that creates a three-dimensional image with the aid of a laser. It was invented in 1947 by Denis Gabor, a Hungarian physicist, who later won the Nobel Prize for his work in this area.

To make a hologram, a laser is used to produce a beam of monochromatic polarized light. This laser beam is split into two beams by a partially reflecting mirror or "beam splitter." One of the beams hits the object and is scattered toward a photo plate. The other laser beam is sent directly to the photo plate and interferes with the scattered beam. The resulting interference pattern is captured on film.

When the film is developed it looks like a meaningless swirl of light and dark lines and the object cannot be seen. In order to reconstruct the image, the film is subsequently illuminated with a laser beam and a three-dimensional image is projected into the eye of an observer. The orientation of the image depends on the angle at which the laser beam strikes the photographic film.

The most important property of the hologram is the fact that every section of the holographic film contains all of the information necessary to construct a whole image. If a small piece of the hologram is used for the reconstruction of the image, a picture of the whole object appears. This provides us with an entirely new way of understanding the order and organization of reality. It is not necessary to cut the whole into pieces in an attempt to study its function. In this phantom-like nature at a deeper level of reality, all things in the Universe are infinitely interconnected. In the holographic Universe the past, present, and future all exist simultaneously.

Working independently in the field of brain research in the 1960s, Stanford University neurologist Karl Pribram was also persuaded of the holographic nature of reality. Pribram explored memory and the brain. The result of his study made him realize that memory is not a direct property of individual neurons, but rather results from the patterns of nerve impulses in the entire brain. In other words, the workings of the brain can be considered to be analogous to a hologram. This theory might also explain how the human brain has the capacity to memorize a huge amount of information in a small amount of space [Pribram, 1984]. Karl Pribram stated that "each organism represents in some manner the Universe, and each portion of the Universe represents in some manner the organism within it" [Pribram, 1982]. Every piece of information in the human thinking process is correlated with every other piece of information, it functions as a cross-correlated system. The brain is able to encode and decode spatial frequencies from our perception into a coherent image.

It has been found that each of our senses is sensitive to a much broader range of frequencies than was previously suspected. If the holographic models of Bohm and Pribram are considered together, it appears that the brain is a hologram, interpreting the holographic Universe.

If our perception can select and transform only a portion of the large continuum of frequencies around us, then what is perceived as objective reality is only a small part of the super-hologram of the Universe. Our reality is an illusion (Maya), in accordance with Indian religious philosophy. We are receivers in the sea of frequencies, and everyone extracts his own physical reality through his own specific channel [Gerber, 2001].

In Nature, holographic properties are illustrated by fractal structures. Fractals are formations where a small part of the structure has a similar pattern as those exhibited by the whole. A river network is an example of a fractal structure. If we magnify any small portion of a river network, we will get a pattern that looks a lot like what we see when we observe an image of the whole river. Likewise, a big branch and a little branch of a tree have similar branching structures regardless of size, as does the whole tree itself. The pattern of ice in a snowflake is another good example of a fractal structure, its shape is made of similar crystallized branches at any level of examination.

To obtain an idea of the organization of matter and energy in the Universe and the part played by our consciousness, we have to study theories of the physical cosmos.

1.3. THE COSMIC THEORIES OF TODAY

Today scientists describe the Universe in terms of two basic parallel theories. One of them is the General Theory of Relativity of Einstein, which includes the phenomena of matter, energy, time, space, and gravity in the observable Universe. According to the General Theory of Relativity, space and time are not rigid. Their form and structure are influenced by matter and energy. A postulate of the General Theory of Relativity is that the presence of matter and energy produces the curvature of space-time. Space and its curvature determine how matter moves. The confirmation of the General Theory of Relativity can be achieved by astronomic observations.

The other theoretical achievement of modern physics is Quantum Mechanics, which includes the study of the ultramicroscopic world of subatomic particles and their interaction. Steven Hawking, in his book *A Brief History of Time*, describes the theory of the Big Bang as the beginning of time and space. What follows paraphrases some of the ideas presented in his book [Hawking, 1989]. An important discovery of the 20th century was made by the astronomer Hubble, who studied the spectra of stars in distant galaxies. He observed a persistent shift of their spectra to lower frequencies, or red side of the color spectrum. From a quantitative analysis of this "red shift," he concluded that the galaxies of stars are moving away from us. The general conclusion is that the Universe is expanding.

The astronomer Friedmann, in an attempt to explain this phenomenon, proposed three possible models of the Universe. They all have a common feature that in the past, billions of years ago, the distance between neighboring galaxies must have been negligible. At that time, in the moments close to what is called the Big Bang, the density of the Universe and curvature of space-time would have approached infinity. From this point of singularity, with a gigantic explosion, time began.

In 1970, Penrose and Hawking showed that at the point of singularity, the volume of space is compressed to zero and the density of matter is infinite. This is the hot model of the beginning of time and space, when the positive energy was at a maximum. At that point, the four forces in the Universe (gravitation, electromagnetic, weak nuclear, and strong nuclear) worked together at a single point. The positive energy of the Universe made matter, and the negative energy resulted in gravitation.

In the first seconds after the explosion, an absolute vacuum appeared and it gave birth to material particles. Particles are created out of energy. Protons, neutrons, and electrons start forming the simplest atoms of hydrogen and helium. From them, through nuclear reactions, other chemical elements are formed.

The theory states that the Universe must either expand forever or contract to the Big Crunch, expected to occur 100 billion years after the Big Bang. The expansion and contraction is like the breathing of the Universe.

The bridge between Einstein's General Theory of Relativity and the Theory of Quantum Mechanics took shape in 1984 through the work of physicists Michael Green and John Schwarz, now known as String Theory. Their idea is that the elementary ingredients of the Universe are not point particles, but rather tiny one-dimensional filaments, somewhat like infinitely thin rubberbands, vibrating constantly. The theory proposes that Strings are ultramicroscopic ingredients which make up the particles out of which, in turn, atoms are made. The strings are so small that they appear like single points on the scale of any measurement. All matter and all forces are proposed to arise from this one basic ingredient, oscillating Strings. All Strings are the same but they vibrate with different resonant patterns. Each elemental particle is a single string exhibiting a different vibration and thus a different energy. The vibrations of unimaginable numbers of strings make up the giant symphony of the Universe [Greene, 1999].

The expansion and cooling at different rates in different regions created variations in the density of the Universe. Gravitational attraction between those regions created a rotation or spin [Hawking, 1989]. Einstein speaks about torsion fields, the quantum spin of empty space, presented in the theory of Einstein-Cartan in the 1920s. The spin and the torsion fields have been studied globally for many years, particularly intensively in Russia (1950–2000). The spin field model of Fermi-Pasta-Ulam (FPU) predicted the formation of nonlinear localized excitations (NLE) with unusually long lifetimes. Their properties are connected with the imprinting of information. The excitations can be roughly explained as little bundles or packets of energy and information. Shipov's theory of the physical vacuum [Shipov, 1998; Kiehn, 2002] presents the idea that the primary torsion field (PTF) appears together with the absolute vacuum and both have the same high energy. This model is the basis for a more general quantum theory, and may explain many subtle energy observations. It might eventually provide a physical theory of consciousness. The Russian quantum physicists A. Akimov and V. Tarasenko envision the human brain as a torsion field [Akimov & Tarasenko, 1992].

The energy in the Universe is summarized in Figure 1.1.

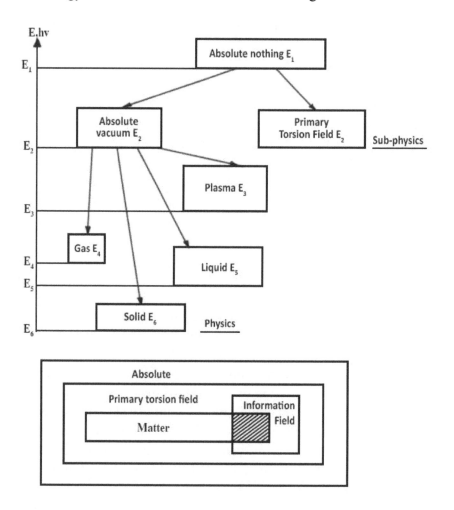

Figure 1.1. The energy of the Universe

In Figure 1.1., the highest energy is located at the point of singularity, E_1. One moment later the absolute vacuum and the primary torsion field (PTF) were born with energy E_2. In the absolute vacuum the polarity of the energy (Yin and Yang, as commonly expressed in Chinese philosophy) already exists. Compression of energy in the absolute vacuum gave birth to subatomic particles. These particles formed the building materials of the world and of consciousness. The subatomic particles oscillate with high energy E_2, studied in the field of theoretical quantum physics.

Later the subatomic particles formed the ions and atoms of the material world. These form the condensed states of plasma (E_3), gas (E_4), liquid (E_5), and solid (E_6) matter, each of which exhibits a progressively reduced form of energy. The properties of matter and the energies E_3 to E_6 are studied in Newtonian physics.

We human beings are made of these material forms. We have the high energies of the primary torsion field as part of our consciousness and relate to the Universe through that field.

It is amazing how similar the properties of the giant cosmic objects and the tiny elementary particles are. The natural properties of live microscopic creatures and those of human beings are very similar. The discourses of the Nobel Prize winner Ervin Laslo convey this idea:

"In the coherently structured and evolving Cosmos the mass of the elementary particles, the number of the particles, and the forces that exist between them are all mysteriously adjusted to favor certain ratios that recur again and again. The living organism is extraordinarily coherent: All parts are multidimensionally, dynamically, and almost instantly correlated with all other parts. What happens to one cell or organ also happens in some way to all other cells and organs—a correlation that recalls (and in fact suggests) the kind of 'entanglement' that characterizes the behavior of quanta in the micro domain. The organism is also coherent with the world around it: What happens in the external milieu of the organism is reflected in some ways in its internal milieu" [László, 2004].

1.4. CONSCIOUSNESS

Many scientists think that: "Consciousness is a nonphysical property that cannot be defined in physical terms" [Harrison, 2003]. But as we saw above, some physicists conclude that consciousness is related to high-energy vibrations in the invisible reality, the virtual reality. This invisible reality is based in the field of energy and information that lies beyond the material world.

Recently, the Russian quantum biologist V. Poponin discovered that a solution of DNA molecules, in vitro, under exposure to weak coherent laser radiation, showed the presence of an energy field. The experiment is named "the DNA phantom effect." The results were confirmed at the Russian Academy of Sciences and at Stanford University, where scientists worked with two different frequencies of laser radiation. It was a laboratory measurement of a subtle energy field. Because it is coupled to conventional electromagnetic fields, the DNA field can be detected and positively identified using standard optical techniques that employ laser radiation. A direct human influence is not involved. The experiment suggested that localized excitations of DNA phantom fields are long-lived. This is in agreement with predictions of the Fermi-Pasta-Ulam (FPU) physical model of the quantum field. This discovery gave quantitative and qualitative support for the development of a new unified nonlinear quantum field theory, which includes a physical theory of consciousness [Poponin].

The achievements of biophysics show that biological living systems form coherent fields and emit coherent light at a steady rate, from a few photons per cell per day or several photons per second per organism. Organisms are emitters and receivers of coherent electromagnetic signals which may be essential for their functioning and their communication [Ho & Popp, 1989; Popp, Gu, & Ho, 1994]. The biophysicist F. A. Popp recently suggested that consciousness be defined as "an active process where actual and potential information are mutually transformed into each other." He thinks that when any cell produces a coherent field, it has fulfilled the necessary condition for consciousness [Popp, 2003].

Our thoughts originate from the primary torsion field (PTF). They are part of the hologram of the Universe. They travel with a speed faster than light, and for them time and distance are irrelevant.

Thoughts are charged with energy and information which react with the primary torsion field (PTF). Thoughts, as physical objects, have wavelike properties and interact according to the laws of Nature. If particular thoughts attempt to act against the laws of the Universe, the PTF can destroy them along with the material body at their source.

I believe that the laws of the Universe include moral laws. We cannot make water go uphill by itself, and similarly we cannot maintain for a long time a lie as a truth.

That which we call our soul is our part of the high-energy portion of the primary torsion field. Our soul never disappears. If our physical body is destroyed, our high-energy part associated with our soul can rejoin the big cosmic source, the primary torsion field (PTF).

Perhaps this source can be called Nature, the Universe, or God. In the 17th century, the philosopher Baruch Spinoza prohibited the equating of God and the Universe. Since we are part of the Universe, perhaps we are part of God.

Everyone is born to create and to develop the big expression of the cosmic Universe. These ideas have been perceived and formulated into ancient wisdom long ago. Buddha said: "In the mind, the mind is not to be found; the nature of mind is clear light." According to the legend, the Egyptian god and teacher Hermes Trismegistus stated that "as above, so below." The macrocosmos is in the microcosmos, and the reverse is true as well.

The stars and the planets are organized into systems that follow cosmic rules and laws. The atoms of the material world are made of protons, neutrons, and electrons, organized in orbital patterns similar to the planetary systems. There is a large central mass with electrons moving in orbits and space between them. The atoms combine to make molecules just as stars group together to form galaxies. Deep in the structure of the subatomic particles, ultra-small-scale building units are found, all acting according to their energies.

A single cell of an embryo contains all of the information needed to create a mature and complete living organism. The cell divides and develops to form the whole body. Likewise, it is possible to take one cell from the body of a living organism and reconstruct a complete organism with its different organs and systems. This process, called cloning, was first used to grow a plant from a cell of an old plant. Later it was used to produce the famous sheep named Dolly.

Genetic engineering will make it possible to produce creatures such as the Centaur of Greek mythology, or to combine genes from a frog and a potato. Such achievements create more questions than answers for science, including serious moral questions.

1.5. THE FIVE ELEMENTS

Creation has its opposite poles: darkness–lightness, male–female, positive–negative. Energy expresses opposition through yin/yang in the philosophy of ancient China and purusha/pracrity in Indian religious philosophy.

For thousands of years, five types of elements and energy fields have been known in the Universe. In Alchemy they are: earth, water, air, fire, and ether. In ancient Chinese philosophy they are: wood, fire, metal, water, and earth. Wood is a symbol of the birth and growing, of turning the passive energy Yin into an active energy Yang. Fire is a symbol of the maximal activity of the energy Yang. Metal shows the beginning of decay of the energy Yang into Yin. Water is a symbol of the passive energy Yin. Earth is at the center and is the axis for cyclic changes. According to Chinese philosophy, man is a functional part of the macrocosmos and is a microcosmos himself; made of the same five elements. The elements enter the body by food and drink, through contact with the environment; and they combine and interact according to the same laws of Nature.

Each of the organs of the human body corresponds to one of the five elements and interacts with the other four. In Chinese medicine, a state of health is obtained through the balance of the five elements. From an energy perspective, Chinese traditional medicine was based on the idea that the essence of health comes through well-balanced opposites of Yang and Yin [Luvsan, 1990].

Yang corresponds to: action, hot, sun, man, hard, heavy, strong, and left. Yin corresponds to: passive, cold, moon, woman, soft, light, weak, and right. Yin and Yang limit each other. An excess of Yin causes a lack of Yang and vice versa. The constant tendency of Yin and Yang to replace each other is the moving force behind change and development in Nature.

Yin and Yang depend on each other. It is impossible to understand up (Yang) if there is no down (Yin). Left (Yang) does not exist without right (Yin), and there is no hot (Yang) without cold (Yin). In this manner, Yin and Yang are the beginning of each other and they produce each other.

The concept of Yin and Yang help explains the structure and function of the human organism. The material part of an organ is Yin and the function of the organ is Yang. The combination of Yin and Yang is constant, the production of one is limited by the other and remains in balance. Pathology begins when an excess of one collects in an organ. The diagnosis is Yang-syndrome or Yin-syndrome, depending on which is in excess.

According to ancient theory, the organs are divided into two types: Yang organs are hollow organs: stomach (E, ST), colon (GI, LI), small intestines (IG, SI), gallbladder (VB, GB), bladder (V, UB), and triple warmer (TR, TW); Yin organs are solid organs: spleen and pancreas (RP, SP), lungs (P, LU), kidneys (R, KI), liver (F, LV), heart (C, HE), and pericardium (MC, CI).

For a continued discussion of the energy of life, I will use the Chinese term chi. Chi is the source of our life; it comes from Nature through radiation from the sun, through food, and through the air which we breathe. This energy, Chi, moves in our body along the meridians. Healing masters found that it is possible to transfer Chi from meridian to meridian. Any blockage of the flow of Chi can lead to pathology. The treatment to such pathology is to remove the blockage points and allow the free flow of Chi once again in the body. The goal is to restore its dynamic transformation, following the cycles of transformation in Nature.

The system of meridians connects the flow of Chi, the live cosmic energy, to any organ of the body. Chi moves in 12 classical, 2 central, and 8 other "may" meridians. In addition there are 12 muscle–ligament meridians connected with the 12 classical meridians. Moving outward from the meridians, Chinese medicine describes more than 170 additional points located on the face, ears, neck, chest, and back.

The five life elements are connected with the meridians as follows.

Wood is connected with the gallbladder and the liver (VB, GB/F, LV); key for the condition of these two organs are symptoms found in the eyes, ligaments, and nails. Anger is also connected with the liver.

Fire corresponds to the heart and small intestines (IG, SI/C, HE); key symptoms can be seen on the tongue and face. The heart determines our emotional condition.

Earth is connected with the stomach, spleen, and pancreas (E, ST/RP, SP); key symptoms can be seen in the mouth and on the lips. The spleen rules the blood and muscles.

Metal is connected with the lungs and colon (P, LU/GI, LI); with key symptom points in the lungs and the colon.

Water is connected with the kidneys and bladder (R, KI/V, UB); key symptoms are found in the ears and genitals. The kidneys rule the bones.

The five elements and the meridians are interconnected.

Figure 1.2., taken from the classical Chinese medical texts, shows the relationship between the meridians.

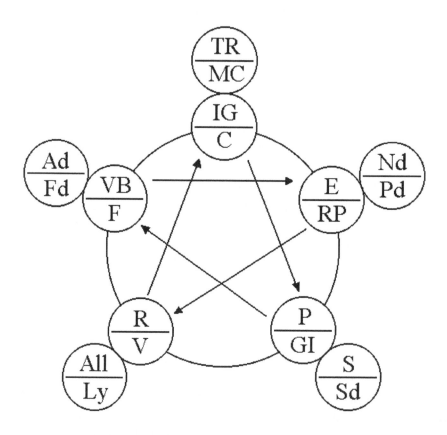

Figure 1.2. U-Sin relationship between the meridians

In Figure 1.2., the generating forces operate clockwise in a circle. Fire helps the earth, giving ash; the earth is a source of metal; metal can turn to liquid (water); water helps the tree (wood) to grow; wood is a fuel for fire. The forces of degeneration are shown by the lines between the elements: fire changes metal; metal can cut wood; wood takes energy from the earth; the earth absorbs water; water extinguishes fire.

According to Chinese medicine, such circular connection is at the basis of the rule called "U-Sin." U-Sin is an important tool for detecting various connected aggravations in our organs. Problems with the gallbladder and liver (VB, GB/F, LV) aggravate the function of the stomach and pancreas (E, ST/RP, SP); the stomach and pancreas (E, ST/RP, SP) aggravate the kidneys and bladder (R, KI/V, UB); the kidneys and bladder (R, KI/V, UB) aggravate the heart and small intestines (C, HE/IG, SI); the heart and small intestines (C, HE/IG, SI) aggravate the lungs and colon (P, LU/GI, LI); the lungs and colon (P, LU/GI, LI) aggravate the gallbladder and liver (VB, GB/F, LI).

The meridians have cycles of activity and periods of minimum and maximum action (see Table 1).

TABLE 1

TIMES OF ACTIVITY OF THE MERIDIANS

Meridian	Hours of the Day with Maximum Energy	Hours of the Day with Minimum Energy
Lungs (P, LU)	3–5	15–17
Colon (GI, LI)	5–7	17–19
Stomach (E, ST)	7–9	19–21
Spleen/Pancreas (RP, SP)	9–11	21–23
Heart (C, HE)	11–13	23–1
Small intestine (IG. SI)	13–15	1–3
Bladder (V, UB)	15–17	3–5
Kidneys (R, KI)	17–19	5–7
Pericardium (MC, CI)	19–21	7–9
Triple burner (TR, WR)	21–23	9–11
Gallbladder (VB, GB)	23–1	11–13
Liver (F, LV)	1–3	13–15

The topology of the meridians is important, but it is more important to accept the ancient wisdom that Chi gives life and the imbalance of Chi creates disease.

Figure 1.3. shows the different energy levels of the system of man. The energy of the physical body is on the basic level while the meridians connect the physical body to the higher energies at the emotional and mental levels.

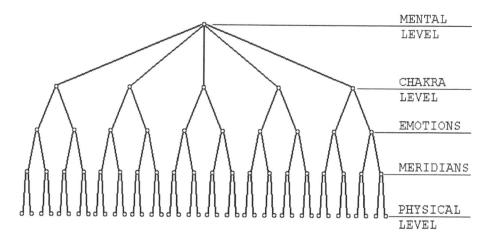

MENTAL
LEVEL

CHAKRA
LEVEL

EMOTIONS

MERIDIANS

PHYSICAL
LEVEL

Figure 1.3. Energy levels of the system of man

In 1954 Dr. Niboyet, a French researcher, studied the meridians. He found biological activity in the meridian points of a dead person. It is recognized that the meridians continue to function for 40 days after death. The chakras, the human energy centers, function for 9 days after death. During these days after death, the Chi structure decomposes and then ceases to function.

In the next chapter I will present the most commonly used points of the meridian system of the human body. I will then proceed to explain their measurements using the Voll method.

CHAPTER 2

ELECTRO ACUPUNCTURE BY VOLL (EAV)

2.1. PRINCIPLES OF THE METHOD

The Electro Acupuncture method by Voll was discovered and developed in Germany by Dr. Reinhold Voll (1909–1988). He was a man with a wide spectrum of interests. First he studied architecture, after that he turned to technical science, studying at a technical university. Later he graduated in medicine.

Dr. Voll became ill with cancer of the bladder. He did not agree with the conventional medical approach. He found the solution to his problem in Chinese traditional medicine, using acupuncture treatment. After that he had twenty years of active life.

Dr. Voll, together with his friend Fritz Werner, an electronics engineer, did intensive medical and technical research into the functioning of the Chinese acupuncture points. In 1953 they found that the physical properties of the human skin in the Chinese acupuncture points were different from any other points on the body. Using a sensitive device called an ohmmeter they found that the skin resistance at any of the Chinese points is twenty times less than at other points on the skin. On the basis of the well-known Ohm's Law:

$$I = U / R$$

where: I = current of electricity
          U = potential
          R = resistance

At the acupuncture points, the following was found:
I = 10–12 μA (Microamperes)
U = 1.0–1.2 V (Volts)
R = 95 kΩ (Kilo-ohms)
Elsewhere on the skin the resistance is about 20 times more,
R = 2,000 kΩ [Scott-Mumby, 1999].

In this way the Chinese acupuncture points, with their low resistance, look like whirlpools, and the flow of the energy is moving from point to point.

After that they discovered that the points could have a resistance, different from the "normal" one, depending on the health of the patient.

The third discovery was made by chance. It was found that by placing an appropriate remedy in contact with the body, the reading of an abnormal point would go to normal [Voll, 1980].

It was confirmed that the acupuncture points could be detected with great accuracy. They are 1–3 mm in diameter. Very soon Dr. Voll realized that there are more meridians on the human body than the number of classical Chinese meridians. He added eight additional Voll meridians to the meridian map and he added some new points to the Chinese meridians as well.

This was the beginning of the development of a new branch of natural medicine, Electro Acupuncture by Voll (EAV). The first machines for these measurements were known as Diateperapuncteur, or Dermatron.

During the 1960s in Korea, Professor Kim Bong Han did a series of studies on the meridian system of rabbits. By injecting radioactive phosphorus (P^{32}) at acupuncture points, he discovered a fine tubule system, following the path of the acupuncture meridians. He found that the meridian system was divided into various subsystems: internal, intra-external, and external. He also found that the meridian duct system was independent of the vascular network. Based on many experiments on different animal species, Professor Kim concluded that the meridian system would appear within fifteen hours of conception and might also play an important role in both replication and differentiation of all cells in the body [Gerber, 2001].

Later, in 1985 in Paris, Jean-Claude Darras, Pierre de Vernejeul, and Pierre Albarede performed experiments that tracked the movement of energy along the meridians. By injecting a solution containing ions of the radioactive element technecium (Tc^{99}), the movement of this element in the meridians was recorded at a speed of about 5 cm/min [De Vernejoul et al., 1985].

In Moscow, Dr. Romen Avagnyan did experiments making acupuncture points visible by using a high-voltage and high-frequency electrical field. When a human hand was put in this field, the points became visible on the skin. The most interesting part of this experiment is the fact that it reveals far more points than are shown in the classical Chinese meridians and even more than the points on the additional meridians found by Dr. Voll [Scott-Mumby, 1999].

Using a similar technique, Dr. Ion Dumitrescu from Romania developed a method, named Electronography, which detects and displays the irritated meridian points. It was found that the points only appeared in electrographic scans of individuals where pathology was present in a particular organ system [Dumitrescu & Kenyon, 1983].

Dr. Voll studied the classical Chinese meridian points in relation to many clinical cases. He found a correlation between the points and their physical position on the organs or their physiological function. As a result he published maps of the Chinese meridians that included some new points and the map of the additional Voll meridians [Voll, 1976]. He described the Chinese meridian points according to Western medicine. In this way he made a connection between traditional Chinese medicine and Western medicine of today. Further, by his findings that homeopathic medicine is able to balance the reading on the meridians, he built a bridge between Chinese medicine and homeopathy [Voll, 1980].

The essence is that a homeopathic remedy, as a source of resonant energy, is able to restore the imbalance of the energy of the meridian. If the remedy has a different vibrational energy, it does not produce any changes in the reading of the Voll machine. In this way Dr. Voll made a synthesis among three main branches of the knowledge of healing and he named it Electro Acupuncture by Voll (EAV).

2.2. MEASUREMENTS

The EAV method is based on the measurements of the specific resistance of the skin at the acupuncture points by a Voll machine. Each Voll machine is a sensitive volt-meter (or ampere-meter, or ohm-meter). The patient holds the passive electrode (cathode) in one hand and the acupuncture points are tested by touching the skin with the other electrode (anode). The device can be digital or analog with a scale from 1 to 100 as designed by Dr. Voll. The measurement is painless and the electrical current of microamperes is so minimal that it is harmless to humans. The meridians must be tested on both sides of the body: right and left. A big difference found between the right side and the left side readings would require special attention.

A reading above 50 is a sign of increased energy at the point, a reading below 50 means a lack of energy. The measurement can be interpreted as follows:

50 is the best reading for any point and indicates a normal condition.

40–60 is accepted as practically normal.

60–65 shows agitation of the point.

65–75 means irritation of the point.

75–85 shows inflammation.

85–100 means high inflammation.

40–35 is marked as the beginning of degeneration.

35–25 means progressive degeneration.

<25 means destructive changes or possible malignancy.

The use of cortisone preparations by the client affects the reading. Cortisone use leads to a very suppressed signal, which could last for several days after the client has stopped taking cortisone.

The reading also depends, to some extent, on the twenty-four hour cycle of the circulation of the energy and the time of minimum and maximum functioning of the meridians (Table 1).

Even though the meridian points are not on the surface of the skin, but in the mesoderm, the area around them is conductive and the skin does not need to be pressed very hard to perform the test. The pressure should be moderate and the same at each point. It is a matter of practice to get used to applying uniform pressure throughout the test.

More important, it is necessary to have a strategy of action: what point to start measuring first, how to interpret the reading, and what to do step by step after that.

Every acupuncture meridian and every point on the meridian can be tested by EAV. The most known and most used are the meridian points on the hands and on the feet. Specific points on the ears (auriculo-points) can be useful, too. Though most corporal points are not used often, a practitioner can utilize a number of them, according to his or her acupuncture knowledge. A phenomenon that Dr. Voll called Indicator Drop, can be observed when the reading reaches its maximum and then suddenly begins to drop to a lower reading. It is an important sign for a pathological process at that point's meridian. Most practitioners of EAV test the Main Points of the meridians only; this is convenient and saves time. However, very often these points are not enough to describe a condition.

2.2.1. THE NECESSARY CONDITIONS

The following conditions for the Voll measurements are necessary:

1. The consultation room has to be free of metal furniture, and the walls and the curtains have to be white.

2. The practitioner has to wear a white overcoat and white gloves.

3. The measurements should be done in the light part of the day, because they depend on the ionization of the air.

4. The effect of any medicine taken the day before by the client is registered by EAV and should be taken into consideration when interpreting the results. If, despite taking medicine for a long time, the meridians still do not give a normal reading, then it means the medicine does not work for the patient's condition and must be changed.

5. Physiotherapy procedures, X-rays, and ultrasound tests are not desirable for three days before EAV.

6. Cosmetics and perfumes should not be used before the test.

7. The skin of the patient should be clean, especially the hands and feet. Moisturizing the skin with water for better conductivity in the area of the measurements is helpful.

8. Metal jewelry, coins, keys, cell phones, and other sources of high frequency radiation have to be removed.

9. The consulting room should be free from geo-pathogenic stress.

2.2.2. VOLL MACHINES

The Voll machines can be manufactured in different ways but their sensitivity and calibration are the most important characteristics of a high-quality machine. Generally, Voll machines are designed to test the resistance of the skin at the meridian points and the effect of a remedy sample for balancing the original reading. The remedy sample to be tested for balancing should be put in contact with the passive electrode. However, the new machines have the signals of a large number of samples in their memory, which makes the use of material samples unnecessary and the work of the Voll practitioner much more efficient.

- The VEGA test machine by Helmut Schimmel (Germany) requires the use of a number of ampules with nosodes for organs, pathogens, and various medicines. The ampules are prepared by Staufen Pharma, Germany. The test searches for an energetically disturbed organ, which may not necessarily be a diseased organ as judged by laboratory tests. The aim is to find the nosode that corrects the disturbance by balancing the energy system of the patient.

- The ELLIS system (Russia) uses a Voll machine for testing and a medicine selector Deta Pharma with memorized electronic signals of many nosodes and different medicines, including homeopathic remedies and remedy combinations from European markets. With Deta Pharma it is possible to test for a medicine and also to prepare all recorded medicines, including combinations. The device is very powerful, and the medicine made by it keeps the signal for years.

- The MSAS system (B.E.S.T. system, Biomeridian, US) is a sophisticated machine with a computer program and a large memory of different samples for testing, including nosodes, homeopathic medicine, and many readymade supplements available on European and American markets. The machine can test the meridians, mark the stressed meridians, offer groups of samples for testing, and make a combined medicine for the client. The MSAS system is registered by the Food and Drug Administration (FDA) in the US.

- The IKG-1 is a Voll machine designed and manufactured in Bulgaria. It was used in my work for most of the research presented in this book. Currently, Biobalance in Sofia, Bulgaria, offers an upgraded and improved model IKG-2, which complies with European legislation for electronic applicances.

Testing with specific nosodes and samples is most important for any Voll testing. The lack of a specific nosode is a limitation for detecting a possible pathogen.

Groups of homeopathic remedies for testing the points of the different meridians are given in N. L. Lupitchev's book [Lupitchev, 1992]. Working with groups of homeopathic remedies instead of a single remedy at a time makes for a more efficient Voll testing process.

We found that it is useful to know the best homeopathic remedies for the different pathogens as well. When the pathogen is known, testing the best-known remedy for this pathogen first will speed up the process. Our research was carried out in the direction of discovering the best homeopathic remedies for the different pathogens.

2.3. WHAT CAN BE ACHIEVED WITH EAV

EAV does not exclude the methods of modern clinical medicine. Proper diagnostic tests are essential and should be considered. The best care for the patient is the combination of and cooperation among general medicine and other different fields of knowledge and methods of healing.

EAV finds that some of the meridians and some of the points in them have higher or lower readings than the normal one. This means that the energy in these meridians is out of balance.

The results of the EAV test cannot be identical with the results of the blood tests of conventional medicine. The blood test measures the physical material quantities such as antibodies, concentration of substances, or different cells. The EAV test measures the changes in the energy level of the organs which can be detected much earlier than the expression of energy distortion at a physical level.

Further testing by EAV would indicate how to reverse the energy imbalance in the body of the patient through an individual therapy. EAV could suggest all of the following items of therapy for every patient: type and dose of medication, combination of supplements, and compatibility of the suggested medicine with other preparations taken by the patient. If a signal for some pathogen appears to affect the energy of some meridians, it does not necessarily mean a diagnosis of illness. In the last days of his life, Louis Pasteur, the father of modern microbiology, said to his friends: "I was not right, the bacterium is nothing, the milieu is everything." Indeed, very often the pathogen is there, but the energy and the parameters of the milieu, the internal environment (acidity, ion concentration, red-ox potential, and other biochemical and biophysical parameters of the organism) are good enough to keep the pathogen under control and to prevent its multiplication.

According to Professor Dr. Charle Nicolle, a winner of the Nobel Prize in Medicine, the "occult disease," or hidden disease, can persist for a long time in an organism [Jadin, 1999]. This is very important especially for the intracellular types of pathogens such as Rickettsia, Chlamydia, and viruses.

However, as soon as something influences and reduces the body's energy (new infection, exhaustion, stress, or emotional problem), it triggers the initiation of a clinical form of this hidden disease.

In this sense, EAV detects the hidden irritations of the energy in the meridians and suggests a way to prevent further complications. This is a preventative medicine, the future of medicine. It has been found that EAV can detect the problem months and years before the clinical manifestation.

Practically everything can be tested by EAV: allopathic medicine, homeopathic remedies, herbal preparations, vitamins, minerals, and other supplements, crystals, liquids, gases, jewelry, animal hair, and many others. An important part of EAV is allergy testing, including foods and many substances in the environment.

The food test is an important part of the work toward balancing the energy of the meridians, a necessary part of the holistic approach to health.

Periodical EAV tests can record the changes in a condition and can suggest an optimization of the medicine accordingly. The dynamic changes of the prescription are very important for a good and fast balancing of the energy.

2.4. CHINESE MERIDIANS AND VOLL MERIDIANS. GUIDE FOR THE MOST USED POINTS

The classical Chinese meridians studied in this book are named according to French and English nomenclature:

1. **Meridian of the Lungs** (P, LU) (Poumons, Lungs)
2. **Meridian of the Colon** (GI, LI) (Gros Intestin, Large Intestine)
3. **Meridian of the Pericardium and circulation** (MC, CI) (Maitre du Coeur, Circulation)
4. **Meridian of the Hormones** (TR, TW) (Trois Rechauffeurs, Triple Warmer)
5. **Meridian of the Small Intestine** (IG, SI) (Intestine Grele, Small Intestine)
6. **Meridian of the Heart** (C, HE) (Coeur, Heart)
7. **Meridian of the Spleen-Pancreas** (RP, SP) (Rate-Pancreas, Spleen-Pancreas)
8. **Meridian of the Liver** (F, LV) (Foie, Liver)
9. **Meridian of the Stomach** (E, ST) (Estomac, Stomach)

10. **Meridian of the Gallbladder** (VB, GB) (Vesicule Biliare, gallbladder)
11. **Meridian of the Kidneys** (R, KI) (Reins, Kidneys)
12. **Meridian of the Bladder** (V, UB) (Vessie, Urinary Bladder)

There are about 370 acupuncture points in the Classical Chinese meridians. An additional 400 points are described in the literature, according to G. Luvsan [Luvsan, 1990]. Only the most important 162 Chinese points are described in this book.

The Voll meridians studied in this book are:
1. **Meridian of the Lymphatic system** (Ly)
2. **Meridian of the Nervous system** (Nd, NE) (Nerve degeneration)
3. **Meridian of the Immune System and Allergy** (Al)
4. **Meridian of the Cellular Metabolism** (Pd, OR) (Parenchyma and Epithelial Degeneration)
5. **Meridian of the Joints** (Ad, JO) (Joint Degeneration)
6. **Meridian of Tissue Degeneration** (Sd, FI) (Fibroid and Connective Tissue Degeneration)
7. **Meridian of the Skin** (S, SK)
8. **Meridian of the Fatty Tissue** (Fd, FI) (Fatty Tissue Degeneration)

All together the number of points in the Voll meridians is about 400. In this book only 62 of the most important Voll points are used. The topography and the description of the points is according to R. Voll [Voll, 1976], N. L. Lupitchev [Lupitchev, 1992], P. Tanev and A. Vlahov [Tanev & Vlahov, 1995], and J. N. Kenyon [Kenyon, 1992]. The nomenclature of the points is given in parentheses according to the MSAS system (BioMeridian, US).

More detailed studies of the original work of Dr. R. Voll [Voll, 1976] could be carried out.

2.4.1. MERIDIAN OF THE LYMPHATIC SYSTEM (Ly)

Ly-1 (Ly-1-1) Throat and tonsils measurement point.
(At the base of the nail of the thumb of the hand, radial side)
Ly-2 (Ly-1-1) Point of the lymph drainage of the ears.
(In the proximal angle of the distal phalange of the thumb)
Ly-3 (Ly-1-2) Control point of the lymphatic system.
(In the distal angle of the proximal phalange of the thumb)

Ly-4 (Ly-1a) Point of the adenoids (nasopharyngeal tonsils).
(In the proximal angle of the proximal phalange of the thumb)

Ly-5 (Ly-2) Point of the lymphatic system of the supramaxillary area (point of the teeth, odontogenic point).
(In the distal angle of the first metacarpal bone)

Ly-5a (Ly-2a) Point of the lymphatic drainage of the eyes.
(In the central part of the first metacarpal bone, radial side)

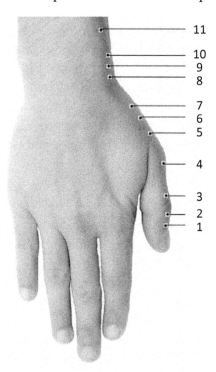

Figure 2.1. Meridian Ly – dorsal side

Ly-6 (Ly-3) Point of the lymphatic flow of the nose and paranasal sinuses.
(In the proximal angle of the first metacarpal bone, radial side)

Ly-7 (Ly-4) Point of the lymphatic vessels of the lungs and the mediastinal lymphatic glands.
(In the anatomic cigarette box between the awl-shaped part of the radius and scaphoid bone)

Ly-8 (Ly-4a) Point of the lymph vessel of the esophagus.
(In the distal part of the awl-shaped part of the radius)

Ly-9 (Ly-4b) Point of the lymphatic vessels of the trachea, larynx, and hypopharynx.
(One cm proximally from the point Ly-8)

Ly-10 (Ly-5) Point of the lymphatic vessels of the heart.
(In the angle formed by the awl-shaped part and the diaphysis of the radius)

2.4.2. MERIDIAN OF THE LUNGS (P, LU)

P-1 (LU-11) Point of the parenchyma of the lungs with the alveoli and the vascular net.
(At the base of the nail of the thumb, ulnar side)

P-2 (LU-10d) Point of the plexus mediastinalis. One of the signs for an asthmatic condition.
(On the proximal phalange of the thumb in the distal angle, formed by diaphysis and epiphysis)

P-3 (LU-10c) Control point of the lungs and trachea.
(On the distal phalange of the thumb, distal angle)

P-4 (LU-10b) Point of the bronchioli.
(On the proximal phalange of the thumb, the distal angle)

P-5 (LU-10a) Point of the visceral layer of the pleura with the lymphatic vessels.
(In the distal angle of the first metacarpal bone, palmar side of the hand)

P-6 (LU-10) Point of the bronchi.
(In the proximal angle of the first metacarpal bone, palmar side of the hand)

P-7 (LU-9a) Point of the bronchial plexus. A sign for asthmatic condition.
(Between the scaphoid bone and the big polyangle bone)

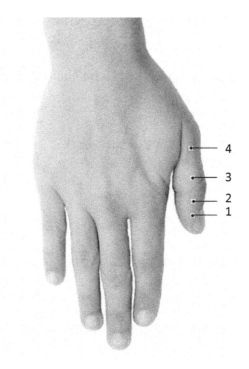

Figure 2.2. Meridian P, LU—dorsal side

P-8 Point of the trachea.
(In the radio-carpal articulation on the proximal fold of the metacarpal bone)

P-9 Point of the upper part of the trachea.
(In the fold of the awl-shaped bone of the wrist)

P-10 Point of the down part of the gullet.
(1 cm proximally from the point P-9)

P-11 Point of the veins of the upper extremities.
(At 3 cm proximally from the fold of the metacarpal joint or 1 cm from the distal end of the radius bone)

P-12 Point of the arteries of the upper extremities.
(2 cm proximally from the point P-8)

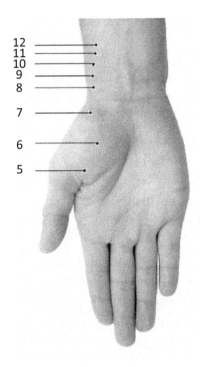

Figure 2.3. Meridian P, LU—palmar side

2.4.3. MERIDIAN OF THE LARGE INTESTINE, OR COLON (GI, LI)

GI-1 (LI-1)   **RIGHT: Point of the right part of the transverse colon.**
                 LEFT: Point of the pelvic colon and the sigmoid flexure.
(At the base of the nail of the index finger, radial side)

GI-2 (LI-1-1) Point of lymphatic system of the colon.
(On the distal phalange of the index finger, in the proximal angle)

GI-3 (LI-1a)   **RIGHT: Point of the Plexus hypogastricus superior.**
                 LEFT: Point of the Plexus iliacus.
(On the middle phalange of the index finger, the proximal angle)

G-4 (LI-1b) Control measurement point of the colon.
(On the middle phalange of the index finger, the proximal angle)

49

GI-5 (LI-1c) Point of the peritoneum in the area of the colon and 2/3 of the ampulla of the colon.

(On the proximal phalange, distal angle of the index finger)

GI-6 (LI-2)   RIGHT: Point of the hepatic flexure of the colon.
              LEFT: Point of the splenic flexure of the colon.

(On the proximal phalange of the index finger, in the proximal angle)

GI-7 (LI-3)   RIGHT: Point of the ascending colon.
              LEFT: Point of the descending colon.

(In the distal angle of the index finger on the metacarpal bone, radial side)

GI-7a (LI-3a) Point of the Omentum majus.

(On the radial side of the 2nd metacarpal bone in the middle of the diaphysis)

GI-8 (LI-4)   RIGHT: Point of the Cecum and appendix.
              LEFT: Left portion of the transverse colon

(In the radio-carpal articulation on the proximal fold of the metacarpal joint)

GI-9 (LI-4a) RIGHT: Point of the appendix with the ileocaecal
              lymph nodes.
              LEFT: Point of the mesenteric lymph nodes.

(On the level of the carpal joints, outside the big muscle extensor of the thumb)

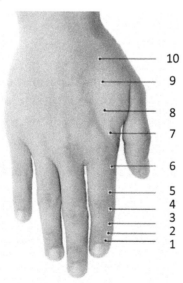

Figure 2.4. Meridian GI, LI – dorsal side

2.4.4. MERIDIAN OF THE NERVOUS SYSTEM (Nd, NE)

Nd-1 (NE-1) Point of the degeneration of the lumbar and sacral spinal marrow.
(At the base of the nail of the index finger, ulnar side)

Nd-3 (NE-1a) Point of the vegetative nervous system or autonomic nervous system.
(In the distal angle of the medial phalange of the index finger, ulnar side)

Nd-4 (NE-1b) Control point of the central and peripheral nerve system.
(In the proximal angle of the medial phalange of the index finger, ulnar side)

Nd-5 (NE-1c) Point of the meninges of the brain and the spinal cord.
(In the distal angle of the proximal phalange of the index finger)

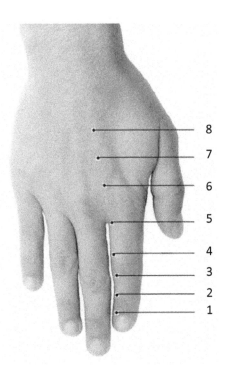

Figure 2.5. Meridian Nd, NE – lateral side

51

Nd-6 (NE-2) Point of the nerve degeneration of the cervical and thoracic part of the spinal cord.

(In the proximal angle of the proximal phalange of the index finger)

Nd-7 (NE-3) Point of the nerve degeneration of the brain and the brain stem.

(In the distal angle of the 2nd metacarpal bone, ulnar side)

Nd-7a (NE-3a) Point of the parasympathetic ganglia.

(In the middle of the 2nd metacarpal bone, ulnar side)

Nd-8 (NE-4) Control point of the cranial nerves.

(In the proximal angle of the 2nd metacarpal bone, ulnar side)

2.4.5. MERIDIAN OF THE PERICARDIUM (MC, CI) (ARTERIAL-VENOUS-LYMPHATIC CIRCULATION) DORSAL SIDE OF THE HAND

MC-1 (CI-1) Point of the arteries.

(At the base of the nail of the middle finger, radial side)

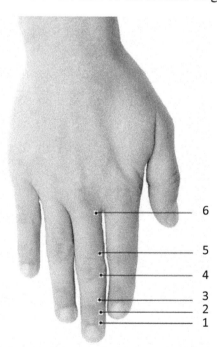

Figure 2.6. Meridian MC, CI – dorsal side

MC-2 RIGHT: Point of the aortic arc and the ganglia of the heart.
LEFT: Point of thoracic aorta and plexus aorticus thoracicus.
(In the distal angle of the medial phalange of the middle finger)

MC-3 (CI-8e) Point of the vegetative innervation of the aortic arch, the thoracic and the abdominal aorta, and the coronary vessels.
(In the distal angle of the medial phalange of the middle finger)

MC-4 (CI-8d) Control measurement point of the arterial-venous-lymphatic system.
(In the proximal angle of the medial phalange of the middle finger)

MC-5 (CI-8c) Point of the abdominal aorta with the Plexus aorticus abdominalis.
(In the distal angle of the proximal phalange of the middle finger)

MC-6 (CI-8b) Point of the beginning of the Cisterna chyli of the thoracic lymphatic flow.
(In the proximal angle of the proximal phalange of the middle finger, radial side)

2.4.6. MERIDIAN OF THE PERICARDIUM (MC, CI) (ARTERIAL-VENOUS-LYMPHATIC CIRCULATION) PALMAR SIDE OF THE HAND

MC-7 (CI-8a)
RIGHT: Point of the blood flow Ductus thoracicus accesorius.
LEFT: Point of the blood flow Ductus accesorius.
(On the surface of the palm in the distal angle of the 3rd metacarpal bone, radial side)

MC-8 (CI-8) Point of the veins.
(On the surface of the palm, in the proximal angle of the 3rd metacarpal bone, radial side)

MC-9 (CI-7b) Point of the lymphatic system of the body.
(On the palm, in the place of connection of the proximal epiphysis of the 2nd and the 3rd metacarpal bones)

MC-0 (CI-7a) Point of the Plexus coronaris cordis of the heart.
(5 mm distal from the middle of the distal fold of the corporal joint)

MC-11 (CI-7) Point of the coronary vessels.
(In the middle of the proximal fold of the carpal joint, i.e. in the proximal angle of the distal phalange of the middle finger)

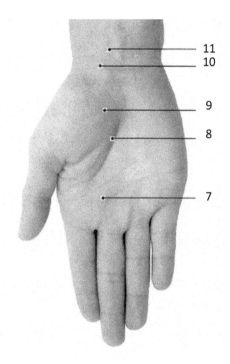

Figure 2.7. Meridian MC, CI—palmar side

2.4.7. MERIDIAN OF THE IMMUNE SYSTEM AND ALLERGY (AL)

Al-1 (Al-1) Point of the allergy of the lower part of the body and the organs of the abdomen and the pelvis, food allergy, and disorders of the intestinal flora.
(At the base of the nail of the middle finger, ulnar side)

Al-2 Point of the allergy loading of the lymphatic system. Useful for testing environmental allergens.
(In the proximal angle of the distal phalange of the middle finger, ulnar side)

Al-3 (Al-1a) Point of allergy loading of the vegetative nerve system. Often shows the presence of parasites.

(In the distal angle of the middle phalange of the middle finger, ulnar side)

Al-4 (Al-1b) Control measurement point of the Reticuloendothelial system (RES)

(In the proximal angle of the middle phalange of the middle finger, ulnar side)

Al-5 (Al-1c) Point of the toxins and vascular sclerosis.

(In the distal angle of the proximal phalange of the middle finger, ulnar side)

Al-6 (Al-2) Control point of the allergy loading of the upper part of the body: chest, neck, throat, upper limbs.

(In the proximal angle of the proximal phalange of the middle finger, ulnar side)

Al-7 (Al-3) Point of the allergy loading of the head.

(In the distal angle of the 3rd metacarpal bone, ulnar side)

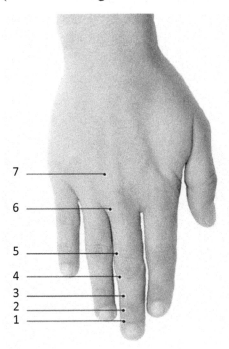

Figure 2.8. Meridian Al—dorsal side

2.4.8. MERIDIAN OF CELLULAR METABOLISM AND THE DEGENERATION OF THE VESSELS, PARENCHYMA, AND EPITHELIUM OF THE ORGANS (Pd, OR)

<u>Pd-1 (OR-1)</u> **Point of the organs of the abdomen, pelvis, and sexual organs.**
(At the base of the nail of the ring finger, radial side)

<u>Pd-2 (OR-1-1)</u> **Point of the lymphatic burdening from cellular or organ degeneration. Anaerobic burdening of the cell metabolism.**
(In the proximal angle of the distal phalange of the ring finger, radial side)

<u>Pd-3 (OR-1a)</u> **Point of the degeneration of the internal organs and vessels and their vegetative provision.**
(In the distal angle of the middle phalange of the ring finger, radial side)

<u>Pd-4 (OR-1b)</u> **Control point of the degeneration of the organs of the body, excluding endocrine and mammary glands.**
(In the proximal angle of the middle phalange of the ring finger, radial side)

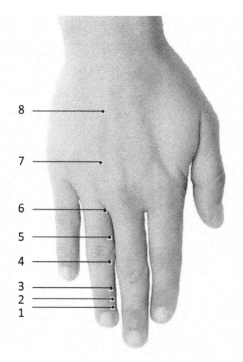

Figure 2.9. Meridian Pd, OR—dorsal side

Pd-5 (OR-1c) Point of the degeneration of the peritoneum.
(In the distal angle of the proximal phalange of the ring finger, radial side)

Pd-6 (OR-1d) Point of the degeneration of the pleura.
(In the proximal angle of the proximal phalange of the ring finger, radial side)

Pd-7 (OR-2) Point of the degeneration of the organs in the chest.
(In the distal angle of the 4th metacarpal bone, radial side)

Pd-8 (OR-3) Point of the degeneration of the organs in the head.
(In the proximal angle of the 4th metacarpal bone, radial side)

2.4.9. MERIDIAN OF THE ENDOCRINE SYSTEM OR TRIPLE WARMER (TR, TW)

TR-1 (TW-1) Point of the gonads and adrenal glands.
(At the base of the nail of the ring finger, ulnar side)

TR-2 Point of the sympathetic nervous system.
(In the proximal angle of the distant phalange of the ring finger, ulnar side)

TR-3 (TW-1a) Point of the ganglia of the cervical part of the sympathetic nervous system.
(In the distal angle of the of the middle phalange of the ring finger, ulnar side)

TR-4 (TW-1b) Control measurement point of the endocrine glands, mammary glands, and the incretory function of the pancreas.
(In the proximal angle of the middle phalange of the ring finger, ulnar side)

TR-5 (TW-1c)
RIGHT: Point of the function of the head of the pancreas; mucous membranes; papillomas and polyps.
LEFT: Point of the secretion of the tail of the pancreas and the blood sugar control.
(At the distal angle of the proximal phalange of the ring finger, ulnar side)

57

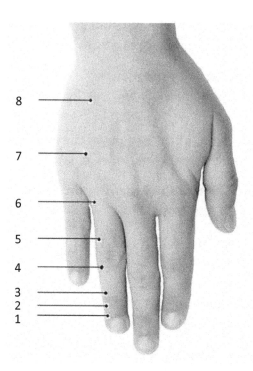

Figure 2.10. Meridian TR, TW – dorsal side

TR-6 (TW-2) Point of the mammary glands.
(In the proximal angle of the proximal phalange of the ring finger, ulnar side)

TR-7 (TW-2) Point of the thyroid, parathyroid, and thymus glands.
(In the distal angle of the 4th metacarpal bone, ulnar side)

TR-8 (TW-3) Point of the hypophysis and epiphysis (pituitary and pineal glands).
(In the proximal angle of the 4th metacarpal bone, ulnar side)

2.4.10. MERIDIAN OF THE SMALL INTESTINE (IG, SI)

IG-1 (SI-1)
RIGHT: Point of the terminal part of the ileum and appendix.
LEFT: Point of the ileum.
(At the base of the nail of the small finger, ulnar side)

IG-2 (SI-1-1) Point of the lymph vessels of the duodenum.
(In the proximal angle of the distal phalange of the small finger, ulnar side)

IG-3 (SI-1a)
   RIGHT: Point of the Plexus mesentericus superior.
   LEFT: Point of the Plexus mesentericus inferior.
(In the distal angle of the middle phalange of the small finger, ulnar side)

IG-4 (SI-1b) Control measurement point of the small intestine.
   RIGHT: Point of the superior, descending, and horizontal duodenum and the terminal part of the appendix.
   LEFT: Point of the ascending part of the duodenum and the flexure between the duodenum and the small intestine.
(In the proximal angle of the middle phalange of the small finger, ulnar side)

IG-5 (SI-1c)
   RIGHT: Right duodenum and terminal ileum.
   LEFT: Point of the duodenum, jejunum, and left ileum.
(In the distal angle of the proximal phalange of the small finger, ulnar side)

IG-6 (SI-2)
   RIGHT: Point of the lower horizontal portion of the duodenum.
   LEFT: Point of the jejunum.
(In the proximal angle of the proximal phalange of the small finger, ulnar side)

IG-7 (SI-3)
   RIGHT: Point of the descending part of the duodenum.
   LEFT: Point of the duodenojejunal flexure.
(In the distal angle of the 5th metacarpal bone)

IG-7a (SI-3a)
   RIGHT: Point of the Papilla duodeni.
   LEFT: Point of the Peyer's patches.
(In the middle of the 5th metacarpal bone)

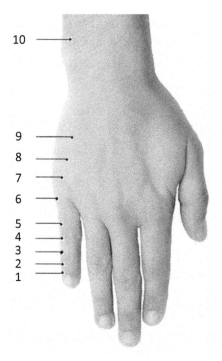

Figure 2.11. Meridian IG, SI dorsal – side

IG-8 (SI-4)
RIGHT: Point of the upper horizontal portion of the duodenum.
LEFT: Ascending part of the duodenum.
(In the proximal angle of the 5th metacarpal bone)

IG-9 (SI-6) Point of the cervical part of the spinal cord.
(In the angle formed by the diaphysis and the awl-shaped part of the ulnar bone)

2.4.11. MERIDIAN OF THE HEART (C, HE)
DORSAL SIDE OF THE HAND

C-1 (HE-9)
RIGHT: Point of the pulmonary valve.
LEFT: Point of the aortic valve.
(At the base of the nail of the small finger, radial side)

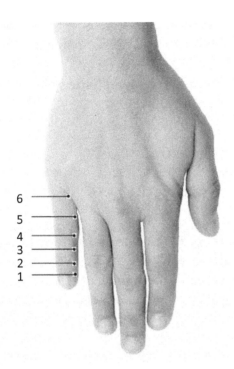

Figure 2.12. Meridian C, HE – dorsal side

C-2 (HE-8f) Point of the subendocardial lymph system.
(In the proximal angle of the distal phalange of the small finger, radial side)

C-3 (HE-8e) Point of the plexus cardiacus.
(In the distal angle of the middle phalange of the small finger, radial side)

C-4 (HE-8d) Point of the lymphatic system of the myocardium.
(In the proximal angle of the medial phalange of the small finger, radial side)

C-5 (HE-8c) Control measurement point of the heart.
(In the distal angle of the proximal phalange of the small finger, radial side)

C-6 (HE-8b) Point of the endocardium.
(In the proximal angle of the proximal phalange of the small finger, radial side)

61

2.4.12. MERIDIAN OF THE HEART (C, HE)
PALMAR SIDE OF THE HAND

<u>C-7 (HE-8a)</u> **Point of the pericardium and its lymphatic system.**
(In the distal angle of the 5th metacarpal bone)

<u>C-8 (HE-8)</u>
      RIGHT: Point of the tricuspid valve.
      LEFT: Point of the mitral valve.
(In the proximal angle of the 5th metacarpal bone)

<u>C-9 (HE-7a)</u>
      RIGHT: Point of the atrioventricular node and the right
            branch of the bundle of His.
      LEFT: Point of the left branch of the bundle of His.
(In the proximal end of the epiphysis of the 4th and 5th metacarpal bones in their joining point)

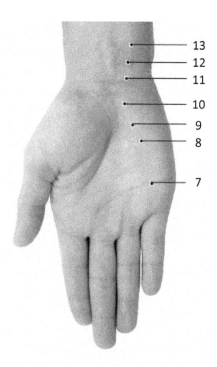

Figure 2.13. Meridian C, HE – palmar side

<u>C-10 (HE-7)</u> Point of the conductive nodal tissue of the heart.
(On the mediocarpal joint between the hamate and pisiform bones)

<u>C-11 (HE-6a)</u>
RIGHT: Point of the sinoauricular node (pacemaker).
LEFT: Point of the nerves of the sinoauricular node,
leading to the atria.
(In the proximal part of the pea-shaped bone on the level of the distal part of the carpal bones)

<u>C-12 (HE)</u> Point of the myocardium.
(At the angle of the awl-shaped part of the lunar bone in the region of the lunar bone and the proximal pit of the carpal bones)

2.4.13. MERIDIAN OF THE SPLEEN–PANCREAS (RP, SP)

<u>RP-1 (SP-1)</u>   RIGHT: Point of the metabolism of the proteins.
LEFT: Point of the function of the white pulp of the
spleen and the lymph of the upper part of the body.
(At the base of the nail, the medial side of the 1st toe)

<u>RP-2 (SP-1a)</u> RIGHT: Control measurement point of the pancreas.
LEFT: Control measurement point of the spleen.
(In the proximal part of the distal phalange of the 1st toe)

<u>RP-3 (SP-1b)</u> RIGHT: Point of the peritoneum of the pancreas.
LEFT: Point of the peritoneum of the spleen.
(In the distal angle of the proximal phalange of the 1st toe)

<u>RP-4 (SP-2)</u>   RIGHT: Point of the purine metabolism,
or uric acid point.
LEFT: Point of the function of the white pulp of the
spleen for the lower part of the body, abdomen,
and pelvis.
(In the proximal angle of the proximal phalange of the 1st toe)

<u>RP-5 (SP-3)</u>   RIGHT: Point of carbohydrate metabolism.
LEFT: Point of the function of the red pulp of the
spleen.
(In the distal angle of the 1st metatarsal bone)

RP-6 (SP-4)   RIGHT: Point of fat metabolism.
         LEFT: Point of the reticuloendothelial system (RES).
(In the proximal angle of the 1st metatarsal bone)

RP-7 (SP-5) Point of the lymphatic system of the lower extremities.
(In the spot formed by the diaphysis and epiphysis of the tibius joint, or on the medial border of the tendon extensor hallucis longus)

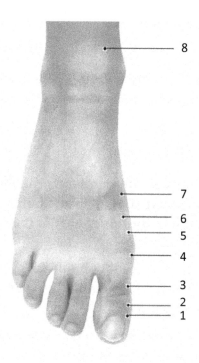

Figure 2.14. Meridian RP, SP – dorsal side

2.4.14. MERIDIAN OF THE LIVER (F, LV)

F-1 (LV-1) Point of the venous system of the liver.
(At the medial side of the base of the nail of the 1st toe)

F-2 (LV-1a) Control measurement point of the liver.
(In the proximal angle of the distal phalange of the 1st toe)

F-3 (LV-1b) Point of the peritoneum of the liver.
(In the distal angle of the proximal phalange of the 1st toe)

F-4 (LV-2) **Point of the liver cells and the lobular system of the liver.**
(In the proximal angle of the proximal phalange of the 1st toe)

F-5 (LV-2a) **Point of the interlobular ducts of the liver.**
(In the distal angle of the 1st metatarsal bone, dorsal side)

F-6 (LV-3) **Point of the perivascular system of the liver.**
(In the proximal angle of the 1st metatarsal bone, dorsal side).

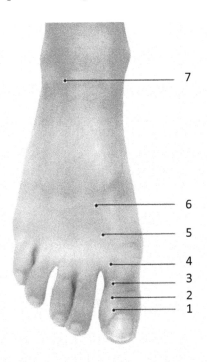

Figure 2.15. Meridian F, LV – dorsal side

2.4.15. MERIDIAN OF THE JOINTS (Ad, JO)

Ad-1 (JO-1) **Point of the pelvic girdle, the spine, the lumbar and sacroiliac area, and the lower extremities.**
(At the base of the nail of the 2nd toe, medial side)

Ad-2 (JO-1-1) **Point of the local effect of toxins in the joints.**
(In the proximal angle of the distal phalange of the 2nd toe, medial side)

Ad-3 (JO-1a) Point of the allergic irritations of the joints.

(In the distal angle of the medial phalange of the 2nd toe, medial side)

Ad-4 (JO-1b) Control measurement point of the joints.

(In the proximal angle of the medial phalange of the 2nd toe, medial side)

Ad-5 (JO-1c) Point of the synovial membranes of the joints.

(In the distal angle of the proximal phalange of the 2nd toe, medial side)

Ad-6 (JO-2) Point of the joints of the neck, shoulders, and upper extremities.

(In the proximal angle of the proximal phalange of the 2nd toe, medial side)

Ad-7 (JO-3) Point of the mandibular joints and the joints of the spine in the areas C-1 and C-2.

(In the distal angle of the 2nd metatarsal bone, medial side)

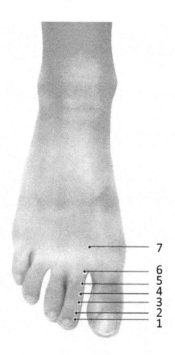

Figure 2.16. Meridian Ad, JO – dorsal side

2.4.16. MERIDIAN OF THE STOMACH (E, ST)

E-1 (ST-45) **RIGHT: Point of the pylorus.**
        LEFT: Point of the corpus of the stomach.
(At the base of the nail of the 2nd toe, dorsal side)

E-2 (ST-44d) **Point of the lymphatic system of the stomach.**
(In the proximal angle of the distal phalange of the 2nd toe, dorsal side)

E-3 (ST-44c) **Point of the solar plexus.**
(In the distal angle of the medial phalange of the 2nd toe, dorsal side)

E-4 (ST-44b) **Control measurement point of the stomach.**
(In the proximal angle of the medial phalange of the 2nd toe, dorsal side)

E-5 (ST-44a) **Point of the mucous membrane and peritoneum of the stomach.**
(In the distal angle of the proximal phalange of the 2nd toe, dorsal side)

E-6 (ST-44) **RIGHT: Point of the pyloric antrum of the stomach.**
        LEFT: Point of the fundus of the stomach.
(In the proximal angle of the proximal phalange of the 2nd toe, dorsal side)

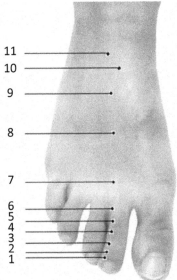

Figure 2.17. Meridian E, ST – dorsal side

E-7 (ST-43a)

RIGHT: Point of the pyloric part of the stomach.
LEFT: Point of the gastric tract in the area of the fundus of the stomach.

(In the distal angle of the 2nd metatarsal bone, dorsal side)

E-8 (ST-43)

RIGHT: Point of the corpus of the stomach.
LEFT: Point of the cardia of the stomach.

(In the proximal angle of the 2nd metatarsal bone, dorsal side)

E-9 (ST-42a) Point of the lower portion of esophagus.

(In the point of the 2nd and 3rd cuneiform bones and the proximal epiphysis of the 2nd metatarsal bone)

E-10 (ST-42) Point of the upper portion of the esophagus.

(In the point of the joint between the scaphoid bone and the 2nd and the 3rd cuneiform bones)

E-11 (ST-41a) Point of the mammary glands.

(In the point of the joint of scaphoid bone, cuboid, and the 3rd cuneiform bones)

2.4.17. MERIDIAN OF CONNECTIVE TISSUE DEGENERATION AND FIBROIDS (Sd, FI)

Sd-1 (FI-1) Point of the Sd of the organs and veins of the lower extremities.

(At the base of the nail of the 3rd toe, medial side)

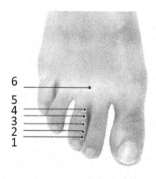

Figure 2.18. Meridian Sd, FI – dorsal side

Sd-2 (FI-1a) Point of the Sd of the tissues and vessels of the genitals and around them.

(Next to the point Sd-1, 3rd toe, medial side)

Sd-4 (FI-1b) Control point of the Sd meridian (adenomas, angiomas, fibromas, lymphangiomas, carcinomas).

(In the proximal angle of the medial phalange of the 3rd toe, medial side)

Sd-5 (FI-1c) Control measurement point of the mucous membranes (papillomas, polyps).

(In the distal angle of the proximal phalange of the 3rd toe, medial side)

Sd-6 (FI-2) Point of the Sd of the upper part of the body, including mammary glands.

(In the proximal angle of the proximal phalange of the 3rd toe, medial side)

Sd-7 (FI-3) Point of the Sd of the organs of the head.

(In the distal angle of the 3rd metatarsal bone, medial side)

2.4.18. MERIDIAN OF THE SKIN (S, SK)

S-1 (SK-1) Point of the skin of the lower portion of the body.

(At the base of the nail of the 3rd toe, dorsal side)

S-2 (SK-1-1) Point of the lymph vessels of the skin.

(In the distal angle of the medial phalange of the 3rd toe, dorsal side)

S-3 (SK-1-2) Point of the allergic burdening of the skin.

(In the distal angle of the medial phalange of the 3rd toe, dorsal side)

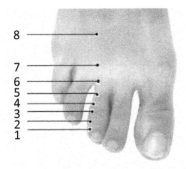

Figure 2.19. Meridian S, SK – dorsal side

69

S-4 (SK-1-3) Control point of the skin and cicatrices (scars).
(In the proximal angle of the medial phalange of the 3rd toe, dorsal side)

S-5 (SK-1a) Point of the scars.
(In the distal angle of the proximal phalange of the 3rd toe, dorsal side)

S-7 (SK-2) Point of the skin of the upper portions of the body.
(In the distal angle of the 3rd metatarsal bone, dorsal side)

S-8 (SK-3) Point of the skin of the head.
(In the proximal angle of the 3rd metatarsal bone, dorsal side)

2.4.19. MERIDIAN OF FATTY TISSUE DEGENERATION (Fd, FA)

Fd-1 (FA-1) Point of fatty tissue degeneration of the abdominal organs and the tissues of the lower extremities.
(At the base of the nail of the 4th toe, medial side)

Fd-4 (FA-1b) Control point of fatty tissue degeneration of the body.
(In the proximal angle of the medial phalange of the 4th toe, medial side)

Fd-6 (FA-2) Point of fatty tissue degeneration of the organs and the vessels of the thoracic cavity (arteries, veins and myocardium).
(In the proximal angle of the proximal phalange of the 4th toe, medial side)

Fd-7 (FA-3) Point of fatty tissue degeneration of the organs and the vessels of the head.
(In the distal angle of the 4th metatarsal bone, medial side)

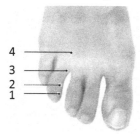

Figure 2.20. Meridian Fd, FA – dorsal side

2.4.20. MERIDIAN OF THE GALLBLADDER (VB, GB)

VB-1 (GB-43d)
> **RIGHT: Point of the ductus choledochus.**
> **LEFT: Point of the ductus hepaticus communis.**
(At the base of the nail of the 4th toe, dorsal side)

VB-2 (GB-43c) Point of the lymphatic system of the gallbladder.
> (In the proximal angle of the distal phalange of the 4th toe, dorsal side)

VB-3 Point of the plexus hepaticus.
> (In the distal angle of the medial phalange of the 4th toe, dorsal side)

VB-4 (GB-43b) Control point of the gallbladder and the bile ducts.
> (In the proximal angle of the medial phalange of the 4th toe, dorsal side)

VB-5 (GB-43a) Point of the omentum in the area of the gallbladder.
> (In the distal angle of the proximal phalange of the 4th toe, dorsal side)

VB-6 (GB-43)
> **RIGHT: Point of the ductus cysticus.**
> **LEFT: Point of the ductus hepaticus dexter.**
(In the proximal angle of the proximal phalange of the 4th toe, dorsal side)

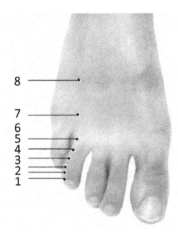

Figure 2.21. Meridian VB, GB – dorsal side

71

VB-7 (GB-42)
RIGHT: Point of the gallbladder.
LEFT: Point of the ductus hepaticus sinister.
(In the distal angle of the 4th metatarsal bone, dorsal side)

VB-8 (GB-41)
RIGHT: Point of the ductus biliferi dexter.
LEFT: Point of the ductus biliferi sinister.
(In the proximal angle of the 4th metatarsal bone, dorsal side)

2.4.21. MERIDIAN OF THE KIDNEYS (R, KI)

R-1 (KI-1) Point of the pelvis of the kidney.
(At the base of the nail of the 5th toe, medial side)

R-2 Point of the lymphatic system of the kidneys and adrenal glands.
(In the proximal angle of the distal phalange of the 5th toe, medial side)

R-3 (KI-1-1) Point of the plexus renalis.
(In the distal angle of the medial phalange of the 5th toe, medial side)

R-4 (KI-1-3) Control measurement point of the kidneys.
(In the proximal angle of the medial phalange of the 5th toe, medial side)

R-5 (KI-1-4) Point of the omentum in the area of the kidneys.
(In the distal angle of the proximal phalange of the 5th toe, medial side)

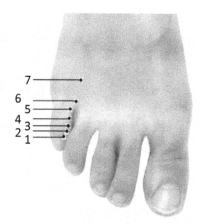

Figure 2.22. Meridian R, KI – dorsal side

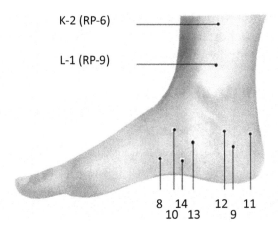

Figure 2.23. Meridian R, KI – medial side

R-6 (KI-1a) Point of the ureter.
(In the proximal angle of the proximal phalange of the 5th toe, medial side)

R-7 (KI-1b) Point of the plexus suprarenalis.
(In the distal angle of the 5th metatarsal bone, medial side)

R-8 (KI-2) Point of the renal medulla.
(Behind the scaphoid bone of the foot)

R-9 (KI-3) Point of the renal cortex.
(On the medial side of the heel bone in the small axilla on the boundary of the surface of the instep)

R-10 (KI-6) Point of the colon, rectum.
(1 cm lower than the low part of the medial ankle)

R-11 (KI-4) Point of the Plexus rectalis medii and inferior.
(In the angle formed from the Achilles tendon and the heel bone, medial side)

R-12 (KI-4a) Point of the anal sphincter.
(In the angle formed from the upper side of the heel bone and posterior part of the talus)

R-13 (KI-5) Point of the anus.
(1 cm lower and further back from the point R-10)

R-14 (KI-2a) Point of the medulla of the kidneys.
(On the cross point of the horizontal line connecting the points R-2, R-3, and the perpendicular from the point R-5)

2.4.22. MERIDIAN OF THE BLADDER (V, UB)

V-1 (UB-67) Point of the body of the bladder.
(At the base of the nail of the 5th toe, dorsal side)

V-2 (UB 66) Point of the lymphatic system of the bladder.
(In the proximal angle of the distal phalange of the 5th toe, dorsal side)

V-3 (UB-66c) Point of the plexus vesicalis.
(In the distal angle of the middle phalange of the 5th toe, dorsal side)

V-4 (UB- 66b) Control measurement point of the bladder.
(In the proximal angle of the middle phalange of the 5th toe, dorsal side)

V-5 Point of the omentum in the area of the bladder and the urogenital organs.
(In the distal angle of the proximal phalange of the 5th toe, dorsal side)

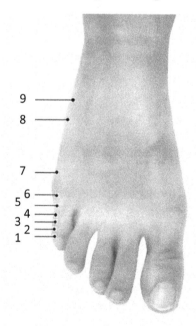

Figure 2.24. Meridian V, UB – dorsal side

74

V-6 (UB-66a) Point of the fundus, cervix, and sphincters of the bladder.
(In the proximal angle of the proximal phalange of the 5th toe, dorsal side)

V-7 (UB-65) MALE: Point of the prostate gland, seminal vesicles, epididymis, penis, and ureters.
FEMALE: Point of the uterus, vagina, and the ligaments of the uterus and ureters.
(In the distal angle of the 5th metatarsal bone)

V-8 (UB-64) MALE: Point of the testes and spermatic cords.
FEMALE: Point of the ovaries and fallopian tubes.
(In the proximal angle of the 5th metatarsal bone)

V-9 (UB-63) Point of the Plexus hypogastricus inferior, important for hemorrhoids.
(In the point of the connection of the bone of the heel and the cub-shaped bone)

V-10 (UB-62) Point of the lumbar area of the spine.
(In the small pit (dimple) of the bone of the heel, dorsal side)

V-11 (UB-60) Point of the nerves of the lower extremities.
(On the backside of the lateral ankle)

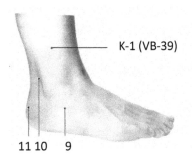

K-1 (VB-39)

11 10   9

Figure 2.25. Meridian V, UB – medial side

CHAPTER 3

HOMEOPATHY, AN ENERGY MEDICINE

3.1. THE LEADING PRINCIPLES OF HOMEOPATHY

Homeopathy as a branch of medicine originates from the work of the German doctor, chemist, and pharmacist Friedrich Christian Samuel Hahnemann (1755–1843). Hahnemann practiced as a doctor for a while and thereafter became a lecturer at the University of Leipzig in the field of chemistry and pharmacology.

While studying the effect of the bark of the Peruvian tree Cinchona, which he used for treating malaria, Hahnemann took doses of an extract of the bark. Surprisingly, he developed the symptoms of malaria. This impressed him greatly. His conclusion was that while the substance quinine had healing properties for an individual sick with malaria, it would cause malaria symptoms in a healthy individual. LIKE CURES LIKE (or *similia similibus curentur*) became his guiding principle for choosing a medicine for treatment of patients. In six years he tested about 300 medicines for their ability to produce disease symptoms in healthy individuals. His book *Organon of Medicine* became the bible of homeopathy [Hahnemann, 1921].

LIKE CURES LIKE became the basic principal in the new medicine homeopathy. For example, the effect of the poison from a beesting is swelling skin with redness and pain, which can be alleviated by the application of cold. These are the symptoms for prescribing the homeopathic remedy Apis, which is made of bee's poison.

In homeopathy the similarity of the symptoms is supposed to cover all organs and systems, and to include the emotional and the mental picture as well. The task of homeopathy is to estimate the total picture of the disturbances, and after a comparison with the properties of homeopathic remedies described in the *Homeopathic Materia Medica* to match the medicine that has the most similar picture.

THE TOTALITY OF THE SYMPTOMS is the second principle in

homeopathy. The estimation of specific and peculiar features is necessary for describing the whole nature of an individual. The homeopathic prescription based on the totality of the symptoms is the best. An ideal remedy (simillimum) is capable of improving all symptoms of the patient. This is what is comonly known as the **CONSTITUTIONAL REMEDY** for an individual.

A crystal has its internal structure, expressed by its shape and form, color, and hardness. In the same way a person has a constitution, which determines his reactions, likes and dislikes, his features and appearance, and his mental and emotional type. A constitutional remedy is thought to restore the person from all types of damage on the physical, emotional, and mental planes. Sometimes it is very difficult to find the best remedy (simillimum), but often something close or similar to it is found (similia). If a remedy which does not suit the patient is prescribed, it does not produce any effect, good or bad.

Knowledge about the action of the substances taken in homeopathic doses is a result of experiments done not on animals, but on volunteers, who were healthy young students in medicine and enthusiastic followers of Hahnemann. Such experiments continue nowadays for description of the properties of new homeopathic remedies. This makes the homeopathic medicine reliable. It really works for humans, on physical, emotional, and mental levels in the way described in the homeopathic literature.

The third principle of homeopathy is the **PRINCIPLE OF THE MINIMUM DOSE**. This is the most disputed area within homeopathy. Hahnemann reduced the doses of the toxic substances until he reached the dilution at which the toxin becomes a medicine. In homeopathy, the choice of the dose is based not on the amount of the substance, but on the reaction and the response from the human organism.

Hahnemann introduced the following dilutions:

1:10	X-potency
1:100	C-potency
1:1000	M-potency
1:50000	LM-potency
1:100000	CM-potency
1:1000000	MM-potency

Here 1 means one part of the original medicine (by weight, or by volume), which is prepared in advance according to a special procedure.

For substances soluble in alcohol or water it is called mother tincture (θ). Solid matter drugs are prepared by mixing the drug with sugar or lactose (milk sugar) and grinding well with a pestle and mortar. The process is called trituration and the powder preparations are called triturations.

The second part of the equation is the weight or the volume of the carrier, i.e. alcohol, distilled water, sugar or lactose.

Another principle of homeopathy is the **PRINCIPLE OF DYNAMIZATION.** After each dilution of the homeopathic remedy, the liquid solutions are shaken and the solid mixtures triturated. The procedure is called dynamization, or potentization, and the remedy is said to be potentized. This is an important procedure because after each dilution and dynamization the homeopathic remedy increases its healing effect.

According to Hahnemann, the reaction between the homeopathic medicine and the human body occurs at the energy level (*prana* in the Indian Ayurvedic philosophy and *chi* in Chinese philosophy). In his publications Hahnemann speaks about the live energy, the vital force, which gives spirit and life to the body and which is not visible, not accessible to our senses. This vital force is the healing power of the homeopathic remedies. He was sure that during dynamization the live energy of the substance enters the solution of the medicine.

Hahnemann thought of the homeopathic treatment as a rational process, based on a relationship of cause and the effect. One of the expressions of this relationship is the existing predisposition to some diseases in individuals. Hahnemann introduced the concept of the MIASM, describing three types of miasm: psora, sycosis, and syphilis. Miasms are inherited influences of diseases that affect the condition of the patient. Often, without any prominent clinical symptoms, they react like a "shade of illness" and make the treatment difficult. Today in homeopathy, tuberculosis and cancer are considered miasms as well.

The **HOLISTIC PRINCIPLE** is another important point of view in homeopathy. A person is an undivided unity of thoughts, emotions, and physical body. The thoughts are the highest level that can be damaged. A damaged thought level can destroy a human completely, while a hopeful, positive, and light thought can make a person recover from a very serious illness. An emotional discomfort or trauma, recent or received long ago, can imprint itself in a person's nature and can affect their spirit, thoughts, and body and can also dictate their mode of behavior and reactions.

In the ideal case one would want to find a remedy that can solve all the health problems of a person. However, a person is not a simple creature and he or she has more than one problem at a time. Social and environmental conditions give us many problems. We live in a polluted environment that constantly pressures us from outside. We need not a single dose of a remedy, but much more to overcome a single condition, and sometimes the individual needs a series of different homeopathic remedies to clear layer after layer of traumas and damage from his mind, body, and soul.

The homeopathic therapy action target is obviously the highest regulation centers responsible for the organism's adaptability to the environment in its physical and emotional aspects. In the human brain the hypothalamus and adenohypophysis act simultaneously as the endocrine organ of the brain where information from the nerves is transformed to hormonal information and vice versa.

Some contemporary medical achievements come close to homeopathic concepts, by means of studying the importance of mental/stress conditions on the endocrine and immune systems. Dr. Glaeser's experiments on students with pre-test anxiety at Ohio State University in the US demonstrate that psychosocial stress could affect the production of T-lymphocytes and change gene function. Dr. E. Rossy confirmed in a report at a medical conference in Garmisch-Partenkirchen, Germany, in 1994, that in response to mental impulses, such as moods, inspiration, and persuasion, the limbic system in the brain affects the biological activity of the hypothalamus, which sends neuropeptide molecules to the blood, such as neurotransmitters, hormones, and immune translators that affect nervous, hormonal, and immune systems. Moreover, the quantities of these molecules are commensurate with homeopathic doses. Neuropeptides are biochemicals that correspond to feelings, a bridge between soul and body.

Dr. Candace Pert, an investigator of endorphins (natural brain opiates responsible for feelings of joy and comfort), has studied neuropeptic receptors on the surface of lymphocytes, monocytes, and macrophages, and as a result has come to the conclusion that the emotional state of the organism is reflected in the neuropeptides and the dynamization of the immune response [Pert, 1997].

Psychosomatic medicine and psychoneuroimmunology being developed in the US over the last 40 years are the bridge between allopathic and homeopathic medicine.

3.2. HOMEOPATHY AND BIOHOLOGRAM

In 1989 N. K. Simeonova, Associate Professor of Pathology at Ukraine State Medical Institute, published an Information–Energy Hologram Theory of the action of homeopathic medicine [Simeonova, 1989]. The author believes that in the process of dynamization the medicine substance molecule goes into a form that has more active electrons. The energy code of the medicine is transferred to the solvent, the vehicle, during dilution and dynamization, i.e. an information–energy field appears, with increasing intensity at each dilution. Every part of the potentized solution keeps the properties and the information of the whole, as in a hologram. The energy–information field passes from one vehicle to another and continues to exist in dilutions that have no more *material* of the substance. The hologram of the energy characteristics of the substance remains, carried by the vehicle.

Being a bioenergy system, the organism too has an information–energy field. The homeopathic medicine affects the human biohologram. In the case of resonance between the two information–energy fields, the physiological system mechanisms responsible for adaptation are activated and numerous therapeutic effects are started in a chain reaction. This resonance affects the nervous, endocrine, and immune systems. This is manifested as endocrine disorders, neurological symptoms, including the vegetative nervous system, and mental symptoms, and functional disturbances such as changes in appetite, sleep, body temperature, and others, have been studied and described in detail in homeopathic repertories for the past 200 years.

3.3. QUANTUM PHOTOCHEMISTRY AND HOMEOPATHY

We realized in 1996 that the laws of quantum photochemistry are very similar to homeopathic principles [Grigorova & Djerekarova, 1996]. We believe that the homeopathic effect of potentized diluted solutions on the human organism energy system is analogous to the photochemical reaction of substances within the ultraviolet (UV) frequency range and visible spectrum. The nature of absorption and emanation of energy quanta in the UV and visible spectral range represents a transfer of electrons between the molecular orbits of substances. The transfers require no special temperature and they are performed effectively enough at room temperature. The energy of these transfers varies from 1.6 to 12 ev, which corresponds to

81

wavelengths from 1.10^{-5} to 8.10^{-5} cm.

The first law of homeopathy, the Law of Similarity, in its deepest essence amazingly resembles the first law of photochemistry, formulated by Grotus in 1817. The law states: "Photochemical transformation is produced only by the light absorbed by the system." By analogy, and this is paraphrased from the energy point of view, the first law of homeopathy can be formulated as follows: "A man, considered as an energy system, can only be influenced by homeopathic substances that introduce a resonant vibration frequency, and which can be absorbed by the organism."

The second law of photochemistry (Stark–Einstein Law, 1912) also assists homeopathy. The essence of it is that only one quantum of energy is necessary and is enough for a photochemical transformation of a molecule. Therefore, there is no doubt that the minimum homeopathic dose is capable of effectively influencing the molecules that regulate function and hence affect the total organism.

3.4. POTENTIZATION OF A SOLUTION AND THE ROLE OF THE SOLVENT

Quantum chemistry is in a position to explain the role of the solvent and the manner of potentization. In the initial mother tincture, the weight of the substance is one-tenth part of the solvent. There are many dissolved molecules hindering each other spatially as well as energetically in this initial solution. Figuratively speaking, they are like vine leaves, crushed and stuffed into a basket. If we pour the basket in the river, we would see how each single leaf floats freely on the water surface, revealing their full shape and beauty. In a similar way the molecules in the diluted solution completely reveal their energy potential when relieved from intermolecular interactions. Then the molecules are affected by the properties of the solvent only.

The solvent role determines the homeopathic action of the substance. Alcohol and water used for this purpose have one common quality: They are polar liquids, including a hydroxyl group ($-OH$) with a free electron coupled to the oxygen atom. This electron couple causes withdrawal of electron density to the oxygen and formation of a partially negative load, therefore the hydrogen atom obtains a partially positive load. Each molecule is polarized as described. The molecules of the total volume interact by "hydrogen bonds," forming a chain of molecules attracted electronically. This could be figured out as follows: Water fills a glass like a metal chain fills a container, in which it is placed. The separate ingredients seem to be placed chaotically, but if we pull up one end of the chain, the whole system will be affected.

The water and alcohol molecules are in a combined state at room temperature and they are released only when heated. This molecule chain tightly envelops the molecule of the dissolved substance and forms hydrogen bonds with it in many places, by stretching it. Thus the molecule is activated, and the electron densities in the dissolved molecule change according to its nature and structure. In the course of electron interactions between the substance and solvent, an energy quantum passes from the molecule into the solvent system, whereas by vibrational frequency the quantum is characteristic of the dissolved molecule. Thus the solvent and the dissolved substance exchange energy. There is nothing strange in this mechanism as this process is well-known in photochemistry. It has been known for a long time that a solution of a luminescent substance gives off brighter light the higher the dilution (up to dilution limits) depending on the nature of the substances.

After drying a luminescent colorant coating on a solid vehicle, a fluorescence of the colorant is observed. The color depends on the nature of the solid vehicle: acid or alkaline. Hence a conclusion is made that the frequency characteristics of the light quantum, corresponding to the electron transfer, depends on the solid vehicle. Lactose is usually used as a solid vehicle in homeopathy, although similar properties are exhibited by sugar. What they have in common is the presence of several hydroxyl groups, which could form hydrogen bonds with the absorbed substance.

The above statement can be related to Simeonova's theory. The molecule of the homeopathic medicine, surrounded by molecules of the solvent, forms an energy system Simeonova calls a "hologram." The main property of the hologram is that each piece of the hologram is a carrier of the complete information for the whole hologram. Similarly, a drop of the homeopathic solution is capable of carrying the information characteristics of the substance into a new volume of solvent, without reducing the strength of the medicine.

3.5. TRANSFER OF ENERGY WITHIN THE DISSOLVED MOLECULE

The total energy of the molecule (E) is the sum of the energy of all possible electron transfers (E_e), the fluctuating energy (E_v), and the rotation energy (E_r).

$$\Delta E = h\Delta = \Delta E_e + \Delta E_v + \Delta E_r$$

The largest share of energy belongs to electron transfers. It depends on the nature of the substance. In the case of the molecule transition from one electron state to another, the value of the energy quantum exactly equals the energy difference of both possible states of the system. Due to absorption of energy quantum, the system passes from a lower energy level E_1 to a higher level E_2.

$$\Delta E = h\Delta = \Delta E_2 - \Delta E_1$$

Acceptance and absorption of energy in discrete portions, quanta, is called quantation. The fluctuating quanta are smaller than the electron transfers quanta, and the rotating quanta are smaller than the fluctuating ones.

We consider that potentization or dynamization of the solution of homeopathic medicine is related to the increase of fluctuating energy of molecules, and hence increase the total energy of the system.

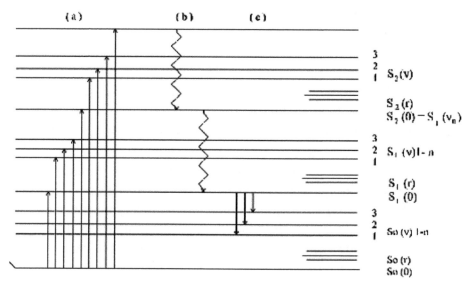

Figure 3.1. Energy quanta transfers in a dissolved molecule

Figure 3.1. shows a scheme, as per Parker [1968], of energy quanta transfers of one molecule of dissolved substance. The following designations are used:

S_o = basic state;
S_1, S_2 = excited states;
$S_o(V_n)$, $S_1(V_n)$, $S_2(V_n)$ = fluctuation sublevels;
$S_o(r)$, $S_1(r)$, $S_2(r)$ = rotational sublevels;
(a) = excitement, absorption of energy;
(b) = intermolecular conversion, $S_2(o) \rightarrow S_1(V_n)$.
(c) = emission, release of energy.

At room temperature an energy quantum is absorbed practically at the zero fluctuation level of the basic state of the system $S_o(o)$ and radiated from the first excited state $S_1(o)$, because the so-called inner molecular conversion appears. After inner conversion, the molecule quickly loses its fluctuation energy when it collides with the molecules of the solvent. Therefore, it is necessary that the homeopathic medicine be dynamized before each use to replenish its fluctuation energy.

The fluctuation levels of the basic state, $S_o(V_n)$, are present to some extent at room temperature. They form a very narrow band of absorption and emission. The absorption spectrum intensity is so weak that it is difficult for it to be registered by a device. The emission band, however, has been confirmed experimentally. Actually, during these experiments it was discovered that the emitted quantum has a higher frequency (energy) than the frequency of the excited quantum. This is a phenomenon known as anti-Stokes luminescence. At first sight, it contradicts one of the basic laws of quantum photochemistry—the Stokes law—according to which the energy of the excited state is always higher than the energy inside the molecule. But this is not a real contradiction because quantum photochemistry gives us an explanation.

We consider that there is a direct parallel between the above-mentioned phenomenon and the dynamization of the homeopathic medicine. The dynamization of the solution makes more fluctuation levels and increases the possibility for quantum transitions of higher frequency, thus increasing the energy effect of the homeopathic medicine.

3.6. THE HOMEOPATHIC REMEDY AS A SPECTRUM OF VIBRATIONAL ENERGY

In this section we continue our discourse about the energy nature of the field formed by any living system based on the ideas of quantum physics. The homeopathic remedy as a source of quantum energy can react with the energy field of the recipient system only if the system needs it.

There are many open questions regarding these ideas that need further investigation. Our effort is directed at tracing some important points and attracting the attention of knowledgeable and honest seekers of the scientific side of homeopathy.

3.6.1. THE CONSTITUTIONAL TYPE

The homeopathic constitutional type is an integral picture of the mind and the body of an individual. It actually describes the manner of a personal response to, and their interaction with, their surroundings. According to E. C. Whitmont [Whitmont, 1993] "Physiological constitution is an organism's unique way of maintaining somatic structural integrity in the face of life's challenges." This response includes the attitude of an individual and their emotional and physical reactions to events and other people.

Our body has about 2×10^{20} cells, each of which oscillates with a specific vibrational frequency. The parameters of the resulting electromagnetic field correspond to an information matrix which dictates the organization and the proper functioning of the whole system, including the body and the mind.

Any decrease of energy by physical influence or emotional trauma causes disturbance to the equilibrium of the system. But the energy absorbed by the system helps it to go to a new equilibrium. In this line of reflection, the homeopathic remedy is a source of pure quantum energy, which can be absorbed only if its vibrational frequency characteristics match those of the energy field of the body.

It is suggested in A. Delinik's experimental and theoretical works [Delinik, 1991, 1999a, 1999b] that the present condition of the health of an individual is expressed in a specific electromagnetic field and that the homeopathic remedy acts by providing specific information to this field. A person's health can be described with their electromagnetic field energy states' intensities as a function of the corresponding spectrum of this field of frequencies (Figure 3.2.).

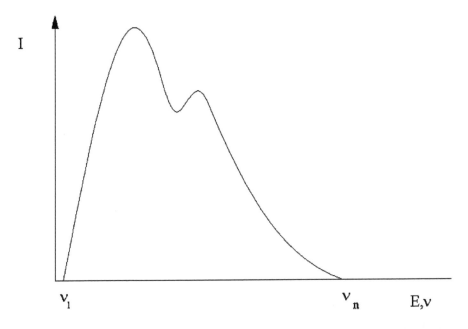

Figure 3.2. Energy spectrum related to the energy conditions (E, v) and their intensity (I)

The energy E and the vibrational frequency (v) are connected according to the relation of A. Einstein:

$$E = hv$$

(where   E = energy of the system
v = frequency of the vibration
h = Planck's constant (6.25×10^{-25} erg).

The spectrum of the health symptoms of a person could be viewed as a spectrum of energy states determined by specific vibrations and their intensity. The interval of the characteristic vibrations ($v_1 - v_n$) can vary. It determines the position of the spectrum on the abscissa (E,v), while the intensity (I) at any point determines the shape of the spectrum (Figure 3.3.).

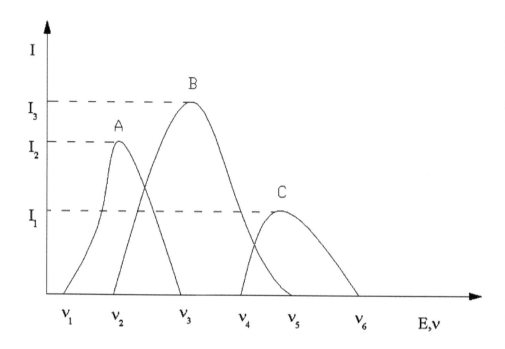

Figure 3.3. Spectrum of the different homeopathic constitutional types A, B, C

In Figure 3.3. the different constitutional types A, B, C have their specific intervals of vibrations (energy) and maximums of intensity:

$$A (v_1 - v_3, I_2); B (v_2 - v_5, I_3); C (v_4 - v_6, I_1).$$

The most energetic is type "C" with a vibration interval $(v_4 - v_6)$ in the area of the higher frequencies.

The effect of the homeopathic remedy on the human organism, considered as an energy system, is similar to the photochemical effect of the ultraviolet frequency range and the visible spectrum on chemical substances: It involves transfer of electrons in the substance's molecular orbits. As we mentioned already, this transfer happens at room temperature and corresponds to the range of wavelengths from 1×10^{-5} to 8.10^{-5} cm. To characterize a specific homeopathic effect on a person's organism, we say that a constitutional type "P" person needs a homeopathic remedy "P". For example, a person with constitutional type Phosphorus needs the remedy Phosphorus. The homeopathic remedy gives the body a spectrum of energy vibrations as described in Figure 3.4.

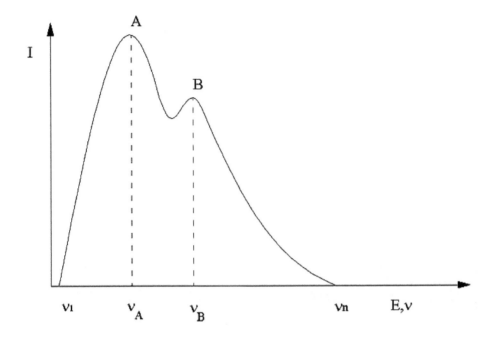

Figure 3.4. Energy spectrum of the remedy AB as a function of the energy vibrations (v_1-v_n) and their intensity (I)

The homeopathic remedy carries the energy spectra of the substance from which it originates. For example, the spectrum of the remedy AB (Figure 3.4.) has two spectral peaks EA and EB in which the intensities of the vibrations represent local maximums (v_A, v_B) in the continuum v_1, v_n.

The remedy AB can be salt, for example, Kali-brom or Nat-mur, or an herbal remedy with two main active substances. The spectrum of the homeopathic remedy could be complicated, with a number of peaks and various vibrations v_1, v_n. A homeopathic polycrest remedy would have a larger spectrum of vibrations, while a "small" remedy would have a narrower spectrum. Table 2 shows the main myasmatic remedies according to Kent's Repertory [Tannock, 1995]. Some remedies are syphilitic and sycotic, others are sycotic and psoric; while sulphur covers all three myasms.

Here the obvious question is: What are the real frequencies of the vibrations v_1 to v_6? This is a very important point because if we know the real parameters of the homeopathic remedies' spectrums, we can

TABLE 2.
THE MAIN MYASMATIC REMEDIES ACCORDING TO KENT
AND THEIR RELATIVE ENERGY INTERVALS

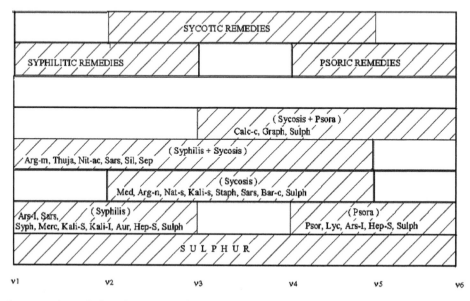

be convinced that homeopathy is no longer an art but a science. We will discuss this later in Chapter 4.

3.6.2. THE POTENCY OF THE REMEDY

We prepare homeopathic remedies of different potencies of the original substance starting with the mother tincture (θ) and then applying a series of dilutions alternated with dynamizations. With each dilution and dynamization, we reach higher potencies. The spectrum of the solution prepared at any of the stages can be described as shown in Figure 3.5.

The mother tincture (θ) contains the full spectrum of the vibrations from v_1 to v_n of the original substance, but the intensity of the reaction of this solution is weak. In the potency 6 CH, we have relatively the same continuum of energy vibrations but the intensity of the reaction of the remedy is increased. An increase of the intensity occurs until the potency is 30 CH. As is shown in Figure 3.5, going to a higher potency is possible, but part of the vibrations fall away. At potency 200 CH, peak B with frequencies around v_B is lost, but peak A has a very high intensity. The use

90

of 200 CH will be effective if the condition of the patient requires vibrations around v_A but there will be no effect from using 200 CH if the patient needs vibrations v_B.

The "M" potencies should be used only when there is an accurate prescription. At "M" potencies, we work directly with the maximal vibrations around v_A. The remedy will work deeply. But if it is not the simillimum, no result will follow.

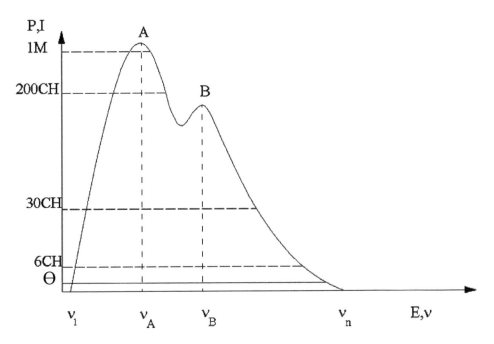

Figure 3.5. Scheme of the different potencies (P) of the remedy AB

The changes during dilution depend on the shape of the spectra of the remedy, and the best potency for a case depends on the energy state of the patient and the vibrations required.

Calorimetric experiments at the University of Athens, carried out by A. Delinic, showed that increasing the potency of solutions of the homeopathic remedy Chamomilla (1 CH, 6 CH, 12 CH, 30 CH) led to an increase in the enthalpy (and energy) of the remedy. The energy structures of the higher potencies of solutions are more stable and a higher temperature is required for decomposition of the structures. The experiments showed that the electrical potentials of solutions increased with the increase of the potency of the homeopathic remedy [Delinik, 1999a].

A lot of scientific research needs to be done in this field, and I firmly believe that these topics will be investigated in the future.

3.6.3. SIMILLIMUM REMEDY

A homeopathic remedy is suitable when the energy spectrum of the remedy corresponds to the energy condition of the patient, that is when the vibrational frequencies of the condition of the patient and the remedy are resonating.

Figure 3.6. presents a spectrum of a homeopathic remedy with three peaks A, B, C and energy interval of vibrations $v_1 - v_4$. The energy spectrum of the patient "P" is completely covered by the spectrum ABC. This is a case of a simillimum remedy ABC for the condition of the patient "P" with the totality of symptoms covered.

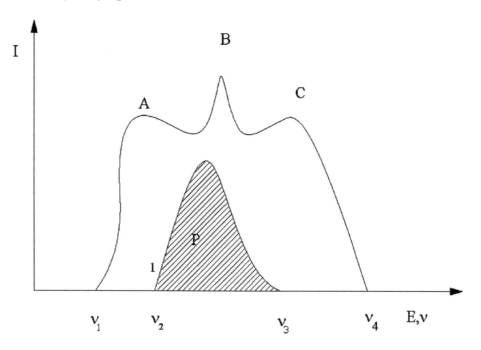

Figure 3.6. Simillimum remedy ABC for the patient "P"

Figure 3.6. shows that of the vibrations $v_1 - v_4$ for a homeopathic remedy ABC, only those in the interval $v_2 - v_3$ are useful to the patient, because those vibrations resonate with his condition. But if the condition of the patient changes for some reason, the remedy no longer covers the spectrum of the new condition P_1 of the patient (Figure 3.7.).

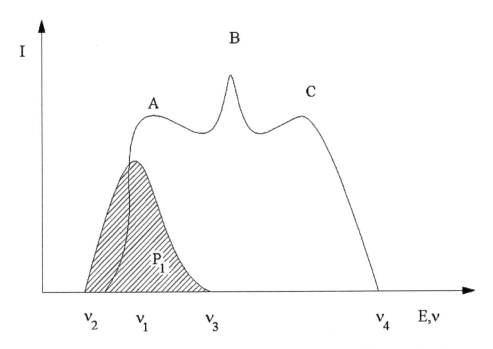

Figure 3.7. The remedy ABC is no longer the simillimum for the condition "P1" of the patient

The remedy ABC no longer covers the interval $v_2 - v_1$. Another remedy with vibrational frequencies specter that includes the interval $v_2 - v_3$ is necessary. A person of a constitutional type "P" needs a homeopathic remedy "P" because the remedy has the closest to the person's specter of vibrational frequencies.

3.6.4. THE PROVING OF THE REMEDY

If three healthy volunteers with constitutional types P_1, P_2, P_3 take part in an experiment to prove the effect of remedy ABC, the experiment may result in the picture presented in Figure 3.8.:

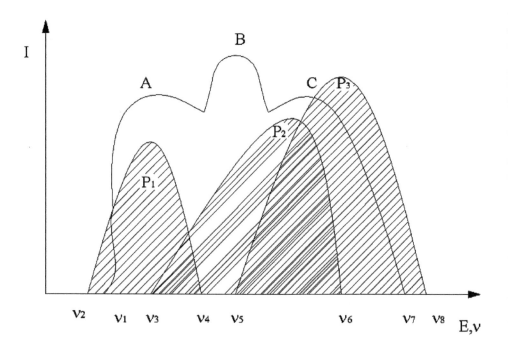

Figure 3.8. An experiment with a remedy ABC and three healthy volunteers P1, P2, P3

P_1: Proved the part of the energy vibrations $v_2 - v_4$ and described the symptoms of the medicine near peak A.

P_2: Proved the vibrations $v_3 - v_6$ and described the symptoms of the reactions near peak C.

P_3: Proved the vibrations $v_5 - v_7$. The symptoms corresponding to $v_7 - v_8$ were not produced by the remedy ABC, so this information was not correct. The information in the area of peak B was not well-covered, so it will not be proved.

If a new volunteer P_4 has no reaction to the remedy taken, it does not mean that he is not sensitive, but it means that his energy condition is far from the interval $v_1 - v_7$ tested. A statistical number of volunteers are necessary for a reliable experiment. And in any case a part of the information is not reliable. That is why at least two groups of volunteers at different times and in different places should conduct proving and then their information can be combined.

3.6.5. HOMEOPATHY HARMONIZES MAN'S ENERGY SYSTEM

In his book *The Science of Homeopathy* [Vithoulkas, 1980] George Vithoulkas presents his concepts about man as part of the energy–information field of the Universe. The cosmic field has a regulatory and form-building influence over a person's body, which is built of proteins and nucleic acids. Health means harmony of the cosmic–human fields' interaction, and disease is an expression of disharmony and field deformation. In such a case, homeopathy has advantages, because as a therapy, it acts at the energy-field level. Depending on the extent of disharmony and the magnitude of the field deformation, the resonant interaction between the organism and the homeopathic medicine is maintained with one or several administrations of medicine. The medicine is the necessary impulse for setting the organism in harmony with the field. For example, the explanation for the action of the nosodes is as follows: Nosodes carry an energy–information code of a specific disease deformation; the immune system uses the nosodes as targets for action and regulation. In some cases the effect is fast and the balance is recovered in only a few minutes, but in most cases sustained treatment is necessary. If we turn to the Mendeleev Periodic Table of (chemical) Elements, we will see that the human organism contains almost all the elements. Some of them are in such microquantities that it is difficult to detect them even by the most modern measuring devices. It is possible that the organism itself potentizes substances taken in with food, separating their information component and sending it where it is necessary. We can imagine that many mechanisms of natural potentization exist in Nature.

Professor W. R. Adey's experiments on the penetration of calcium ions into the brains of rabbits show that the maximum amount of calcium enters when an electromagnetic field with a specific frequency is applied at a low intensity. These frequencies and intensities correspond to biological and physical conditions that satisfy the needs of the organism and are called the "window of Adey" [Adey, 1988]. The system reacts and accepts only substances and electromagnetic fields suitable for its present energy condition.

The ideas proposed above can be illustrated with one practical case, in which it is important to notice that the increase in the general energy of the patient's system directly correlates to improvement in her emotional and physical condition.

Case: Roxanne, 18 months old

The child presented red and dry eczema—big patches on the legs and arms, worse on the right side. The eczema began when she was nine months old; previous to that, she had a bad diaper rash. Roxanne was thin, with dark eyes, dark hair, and a pale face. She was irritable and violent. She did not allow me to touch her or even to look at her. She wanted to strike her mother, she refused to be seen by me, so I had to do Voll tests through her mother's body. I gave her a doll to play with and she immediately tore off the doll's dress. The mother explained that the child preferred to be naked at home.

She had poor appetite. She was restless at night, too: She would wake up several times and then not want to go back to sleep. In general, she was a nervous and restless child. She caught cold easily and had recurrent respiratory tract infections with a clear to yellow discharge with bloody strings in it sometimes. She liked fresh air and she was better at the seaside.

I saw her four times within six months: I – 1 November 1999; II – 19 November 1999; III – 25 February 2000; IV – 26 April 2000. Allergy testing by EAV (Electro Acupuncture by Voll) was done during the first visit. The following allergens were determined: dairy products, soy, beans, red meat, chicken meat, peanuts, cashew nuts, sugar, rice, eggplant, and onions. I suggested that the mother stop giving her these allergenic foods for three months.

Rx: Two remedies were recommended: Remedy No. 1 – Hyosciamus 30 CH (×1 dose a day for 6 days); after that Remedy No. 2 to be given – Medorrhinum 200 CH (×1 dose a day for 6 days).

Second visit, 3 weeks later: The eczema was better. The child was seen because she had swollen glands. The child was still on the diet.

Rx: Merc-Iod-Flav 6 CH (3× 1 dose for two weeks; after that to repeat the two remedies given first and to take Dynajets vitamins for children (×1 tablet a day).

Third visit, 2 months later: The skin had cleared completely. She remained on the diet. The swollen glands had subsided. The mother found that if the child ate sugar, a small swollen spot would appear like a bag under the right eye. The child was much calmer now and would allow me to speak to her. When I did this she smiled. She was not wild any longer. The mother told me that she was now a different child. She was now attached to her mother and she wanted her to be present all through the night. The reason for the visit was that Roxanne was coughing and had a green discharge from the nose. Allergy testing by EAV: Allergens were only chicken, meat, and sugar.

Rx: Pulsatilla 30 CH (2× 1 dose a day) and Drosinulla cough syrup (1/2 teaspoon × 3–4 a day)

The next visit was 2 months later. The child was very well. The skin was clear.

In this case we have the following progression of remedies:

Hyosciamus → Medorrhinum → Merc–Iod–Flav → Pulsatilla,

with improvement of the vital energy of the child, which was manifested as mood improvement, allergies reduction, and cleared skin. This case showed a typical development according to Dr. Herscu's [Herscu, 1996] hierarchy of homeopathic remedies' prescription progression in children. The most difficult types of children are described in phase IV as they need Hyosciamus, Tarentulla, and Veratrum album in this order. The condition during phase II requires homeopathic nosodes, in this case Medorrhinum.

After that, the most common phase I basic group of remedies for children includes: Calcarea carbonica, Lycopodium, Natrium muriaticum, Phosphorus, Pulsatilla, and Sulphur [Herscu, 1996]. The energy spectrum of the remedies used in the case of Roxanne are described in Figure 3.9.

We do not know the spectral vibrations of these remedies, and we can only guess that the remedies for difficult children in Dr. Herscu's system show lower energy than the common constitutional remedies for children.

The following conclusions can be made for the action of homeopathy:

1. The constitution of an individual has an energy spectrum, sensitive to various environmental influences.

2. The homeopathic remedy has a spectrum of energy released by the original substance.

3. The remedies have different energy spectra, specific vibration frequencies, and intensities.

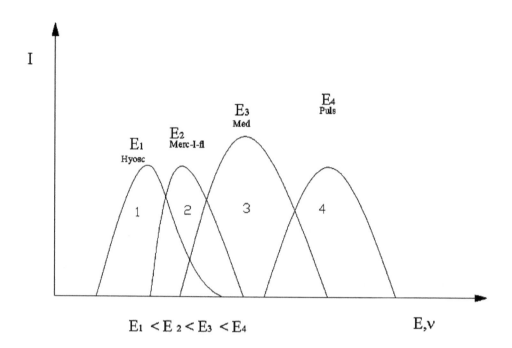

$$E_1 < E_2 < E_3 < E_4$$

Figure 3.9. Scheme of the improvement of the vital energy of a child, from Hyosciamus to Pulsatilla

4. A simillimum remedy has an identical or a wider spectrum of frequencies than those of the disease.

5. The energy system of the body can only respond to the quanta of matching frequencies of the remedy with which it resonates.

6. Homeopathy acts by harmonizing the energy field and increasing the general energy of the human system.

An important task of homeopathy today is to search for experimental verification of the homeopathic medicine's energy action. Only then will homeopathy be accepted as an exact science of the 21st century and not just an art of medical treatment.

3.7. THE ART AND THE SCIENCE OF HOMEOPATHY

Homeopathy has principles that make it unique. It is a gentle medicine working with the subtle energies of man. This is the medicine that considers man in his/her entirety: body, mind, and spirit, and when he is ill it does not treat him as if he is a broken machine.

Homeopathic remedies are a fantastic tool. They are a real miracle: pure energy, given in fine portions, absorbed by the systems that control the regulatory functions of the body. Why has homeopathy not been accepted more widely during its 200 years of development? Why do the skeptics think that homeopathic medicine works only due to a placebo effect? Homeopathy works if the right remedy is found. But the right remedy is often not found. The homeopath has to be really skilled to have consistent success. It is a real art to pick out all the symptoms, to describe the modalities of the symptoms, and to combine them into a total picture, characteristic of that patient. After that, it is necessary to compare this picture of the patient with pictures of different homeopathic medicines, described in the books of the *Materia Medica*. The comparison is based on the subjective estimation of the homeopath. His individuality will be imprinted on the objective assessment. The prescribed medicine may work well or may not.

At present homeopathy has no scientific theoretical explanation for the action of homeopathic medicines. This gives the skeptics reason to say that homeopathy is not based on science. Homeopathy will remain only an art as long as the physical effects of the action of the remedies have not been described and the energy spectra of the remedies are unknown. That is why it is most important for the development of homeopathy not to test new medicines, but to use the great achievements of modern science to understand and explain the theory of homeopathy as it is already practiced.

Such a modern technical method is EAV. It shows the condition of the organs and the systems before and after testing a homeopathic remedy, and it can easily show if the medicine has worked or not. The combination of the knowledge of traditional Chinese medicine, the knowledge of general medicine, and the use of homeopathic remedies will contribute to the development of a gentle and humane future medicine. I believe that homeopaths should not be afraid to look beyond the mainstream of homeopathy. Scientific techniques and computer information technologies are developing fast and they can help homeopathy if these new achievements are used on its behalf.

CHAPTER 4

THE EAV METHOD AS A SUPPORT FOR HOMEOPATHY

The Voll method of testing the effectiveness of substances such as vitamins, minerals, herbal medicine, and homeopathic remedies in the treatment of different health conditions, could be used for the further development of homeopathy. The following points outline the field of research that has been done for proving the power of homeopathy.

1. The effects of some homeopathic remedies on patients affected by pathogenic bacteria were recorded. This showed how gentle homeopathic remedies could fight some pathogens that are resistant to many antibiotics.

2. The spectral frequencies of some homeopathic remedies were determined through comparison with the resonance frequencies of different pathogens.

3. Fungal infections and their homeopathic treatments were recorded.

4. Homeopathic remedies for viral infections were found and proved.

5. Homeopathic remedies for balancing the bacterial flora of the bowels and the relationship between allergy, pathogenic bowel flora, and disturbances of the function of the digestive system were found.

6. The specific reaction to some homeopathic remedies of different organs was studied and the confirmation of their role as "organ remedies" was carried out. This included their role for normalizing the physiological function of the organs and for detoxification or drainage.

7. The competitiveness of two or more homeopathic remedies was tested. This study was not done to revise the table of Kent [Kent, 1996], but to find the combination of remedies that was most effective for each client.

8. The interactions of homeopathic remedies, vitamins, minerals, and other supplements were observed. These interactions are important to note, because most clients take supplements all the time.

9. The effects of homeopathic nosodes and their resonance vibrations as a treatment method were recorded.

10. The effects of homeopathic medicine in different potencies were tested.

11. The effects of specific diets on pathogenic bacterial flora during homeopathic treatment were discovered.

12. The effects of homeopathic medicine on parasitic infestations were confirmed.

The EAV method, used for research in the field of homeopathy, made the results measurable and repeatable, both necessary conditions for any scientific work. Our EAV-enabled research was directed at fulfilling the above plan. Not everything in the plan was carried out, but the results showed that research in the field of homeopathy could be done even with a simple technical device such as the Voll machine.

The steps followed with each client were as follows:

First the client was tested so as to describe the condition of the organs and systems.

The second task was to find whether any pathogen was responsible for the disturbance of the system. The disturbance could be, for example, due to the presence of parasites, bacteria, fungi, viruses, Rickettsia, or Chlamydia infection. Sometimes it could be a functional disorder of some organ or system.

The third task was to find a remedy or combination of remedies to balance the meridian system(s).

After that a food test was done. It was suggested to the client that any food that was shown to irritate the immune system be avoided for three months.

The results obtained from successful cases were collected in the following tables (which are in the Appendix):

Table 3. Bacterial and fungal pathogens and homeopathic remedies confirmed by EAV tests as specific for these pathogens

EAV practitioners could use the information from Table 3 for finding homeopathic medicines that balance the meridians. This information could be loaded as custom library files into computer systems such as the MSAS system by BioMeridian used by EAV practitioners.

Homeopaths could also use these results and could add them to Homeopathic Medical Repertories after they are confirmed by other independent tests.

Table 4. Bacterial and fungal pathogens related to food intolerance

These results could be used to guide the practitioner to quickly identify specific bacterial and fungal pathogens for testing the patient for food intolerance. One interesting finding from our tests is that while allergens are specific to every patient, most allergic reactions originate from pathogens in the intestines.

Table 5. Some viruses and homeopathic remedies specific for them as proved by EAV tests

This data could be useful for homeopaths as well as for EAV practitioners. Any type of medicine offered to fight viruses deserves attention nowadays.

Table 6. Homeopathic remedies active for different pathogens and their resonance frequencies

These results could be interesting for homeopaths. They assist in determining the homeopathic remedies' spectral areas of action.

Many more pathogens could be added to Tables 3 to 6 as more and more remedies undergo further research. Additional research will also help determine the shape of the homeopathic remedies spectra in more detail.

Some of the results of Table 6 are presented in graphic form. Figures 4.1. to 4.6. show schematically the frequency intervals characteristic for some homeopathic remedies. The intensities and the real shape of their spectra have not been determined yet. A good research project could be done, for example, on the spectral intervals of the resonance frequencies of pathogens as recorded by R. R. Rife on his resonator machine.

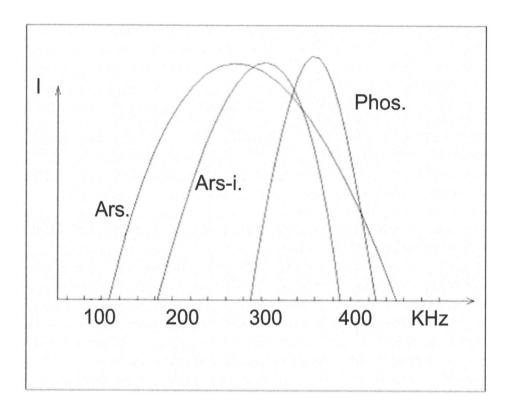

Figure 4.1. The spectral areas of homeopathic remedies
Arsenicum album, Arsenicum iodatum, and Phosphorus:
Ars. (128–420 KHz), Ars-i. (184–396 KHz), Phos. (288–434 KHz)

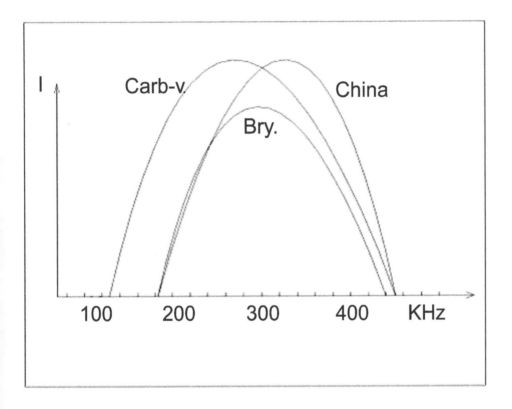

Figure 4.2. The spectral areas of the homeopathic remedies
Carbo vegetabilis, Bryonia, and China:
Carb-v. (128-442 KHz), Bry. (184-420 KHz), China (184-442 KHz)

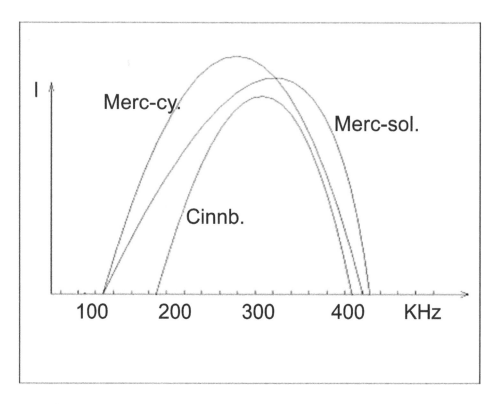

Figure 4.3. The spectral areas of three homeopathic remedies from the group of Mercury salts:
Mercurius cyanatus (128–418 KHz), Cinnabaris (184–409 KHz), Mercurius solubilis (128–434 KHz)

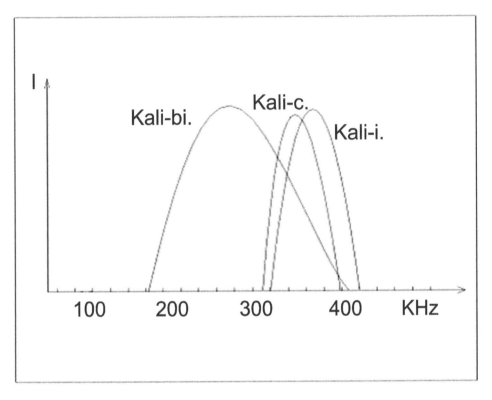

Figure 4.4. The spectral areas of three homeopathic remedies from the group of Potassium salts:
Kalium bichromicum (362–396 KHz),
Kalium carbonicum (318–396 KHz),
Kalium iodatum (323–420 KHz)

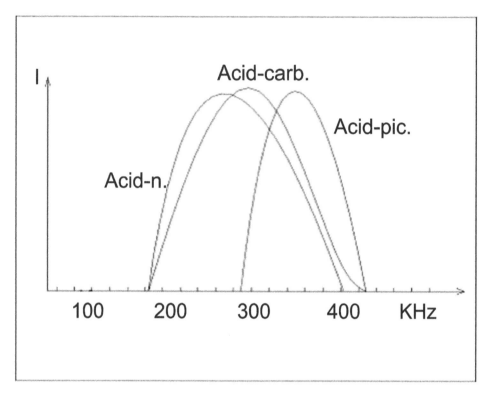

Figure 4.5. The spectral areas of three homeopathic remedies from the Acidic group:
Acidum nitricum (184–413 KHz),
Acidum carbolicum (184–420),
Acidum picricum (288–396 KHz)

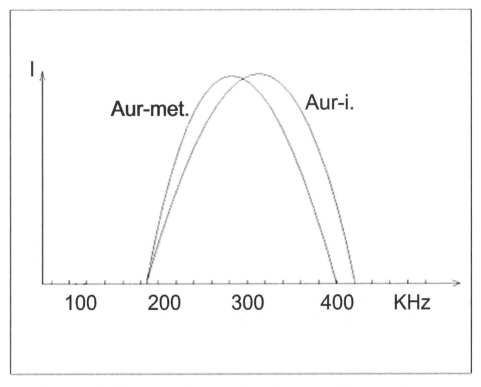

Figure 4.6. The spectral areas of the homeopathic remedies
Aurum metalicum and Aurum iodatum:
Aur-met. (184–413 KHz), Aur-i. (184–420 KHz)

A homeopathic remedy effect on a pathogen can be predicted from the remedy and the pathogen's known spectral intervals. For example, fungi have low-resonance frequencies, therefore the best homeopathic remedies for them are Acidum carbolicum, Acidum floricum, Acidum nitricum, and Aurums, which, too, have low-resonance frequencies. The experimental results confirm that these homeopathic remedies are indeed powerful for treating fungal infections.

The treatment effects of some homeopathic remedies on parasites are summarized in Table 7. From a practical point of view, these results are useful for clearing parasites and supporting the immune system homeopathically. From a theoretical point of view, knowing that the family of the parasites have an energy bandwidth of about 350 to 500 KHz, we can draw conclusions about the spectra of such remedies.

The fact that the homeopathic remedies can work not only for microscopic parasites but also for much larger ones shows that the quantum energy supplied by the remedy is powerful enough to restore the balance of the meridian system destroyed by the function of the parasite (Table 7).

Different approaches can be invented for research in this field. However, knowledge and inspiration together with hard work are the most important drivers of the development of homeopathy. A more detailed description of the pathogens and the EAV tests for them are presented in the following Chapter 5.

CHAPTER 5

EAV AND HOMEOPATHY IN PRACTICE

5.1. ALLERGY TESTING BY EAV

The term *allergy* applies to the adverse reactions of an individual to substances such as foods, beverages, chemicals, and vegetable and animal matter. Any allergy or other abnormal physiological reaction is an expression of the individual's energy system disturbance from some kind of environmental agent's exposure. These agents can be exotoxins (food, air, chemicals, radiation) and endotoxins (toxins produced by pathogens, toxins from metabolized food, and medications or the products of our biochemistry in the case of poor elimination).

5.1.1. THE MOST COMMON MANIFESTATIONS OF ALLERGY

Hay fever is a seasonal allergic reaction, associated with mold spores, tree pollens, grasses, and flowers. It depends on the temperature and the humidity of the air and it usually increases in spring and summer. Hay fever is expressed as sneezing, burning, and watery eyes, runny nose, swelling of the face, and irritation of the throat.

Allergic rhinitis involves hay fever, but is very often not a seasonal problem. The allergy cause could be animal fur, dandruff, house dust, mites, feathers, mold spores, chemicals, fumes from industry, and any substances in the house or in the working environment. An important cause of allergic rhinitis is food. For many people, sugar and dairy products appear to be mucous-producing. In chronic cases, eliminating some common foods from the diet is a necessary allergy treatment step.

Ear infections, sinusitis, and persistent postnasal drip are often related to allergic rhinitis. The change of milk or formula to a different one can sometimes improve the chronic ear infection condition in an infant.

111

Dairy products, sugar, bread, and alcohol are the most common underlying causes of these problems in adults. However, sometimes a chronic infection caused by pathogens can be the persistent cause of all of the allergy symptoms, and it is essential to test for bacterial or viral pathogens.

Asthma is the result of a chronic inflammation of the bronchial airways. The bronchial walls swell, become narrow and obstructed, even constricted. Various white blood cells, such as lymphocytes, neutrophils, eosinophils, and mast cells react to the allergen and cause the inflammation. Asthma attacks can be triggered by a number of factors such as cold air, smoke, exercising, other infections, stress, and medications. Asthmatic breathing is difficult, with much wheezing, and the attack can be dramatic.

Asthma is often related to allergy, but not every case of asthma is caused by allergy. There are cases related to different bacterial or fungal infections, most often Candida, Mycoplasma, Klebsiella, Staphylococcus, or other chronic bacterial infections. It is essential to test infants for parasites. In any case of asthma it is necessary to do a proper allergy test for foods, grasses, pollens, and other environmental allergens. The test for asthma is done on the meridians of the immune and lymphatic systems, (Al, Ly), lungs (P/LU), pancreas and spleen (RP/SP), liver (F/LI), and intestines (GI/LV, IG/SI).

Eye irritation manifested as redness, and itchy and watery eyes can be a sign of an allergic reaction. However, it is advisable to visit an ophthalmologist in any cases involving complaints with the eyes. Sometimes the condition may be much more serious than allergy.

Urticaria (hives) is often allergy-related. In some cases it could be a serious allergic reaction. It is usually expressed as swollen spots, like groups of insect bites, on the skin. If it is accompanied by swollen lips, tongue, or throat, it should be seriously treated, even including hospitalization. This is because if it continues for a long time it can be the beginning of a possible anaphylactic shock. Once out of danger, though, thorough allergy and organ tests must be done. In the case of chronic urticaria, it is important to find the source of the toxins in the system. Drugs, foods, and contact with some toxic substances can all cause recurring urticaria. Also in the urticaria group are allergies to cold, sunlight, heat, or pressure.

Eczema is the general name for one of the most commonplace allergy-related skin problems. The skin can have dry, peeling, itchy, red, or crusty patches. Neurodermatitis, contact dermatitis, atopic dermatitis, and other related forms need the same testing and the same approach to healing. Asthma, eczema, and allergic rhinitis are usually connected. Suppression of one of them increases the others. For this reason, the use of cortisone preparations can improve the condition, but cannot be the solution to the problem. Finding the source of the toxins in the system and using special procedures and a proper diet to clean and keep them out of the system are more natural approaches to healing. In the case of eczema, a full test for food allergies is essential.

Food allergy

According to the formulations of the American Academy of Allergy and Immunology (1986), there are several types of allergies and sensitivities to food [Joung, Dobozin, & Miner, 1999]:
- Adverse reactions to food or food additives and all untoward reactions to food.
- Food allergy or hypersensitivity to food includes reactions involving the immune system.
- Anaphylaxis—severe systemic reactions that can be fatal.
- Food intolerance includes any abnormal response to food that is not mediated by the immune system.
- Food poisoning or toxicity is any reaction to bacteria and their toxins or to chemicals in food.
- Pharmacological reactions are reactions to substances acting as drugs, for example caffeine. Many substances used as medications can cause allergic reactions.
- Metabolic food disorders are caused by the inability to metabolize a given food, for example lactose intolerance.
- Reactions of sensitivity unrelated to allergies.

Food-related reactions are common. The intake of good quality food is most important for proper building of our organisms. It helps to keep the friendly gut bacteria in good condition and the immune system out of persistent stress. Real client cases show that most of the allergic reactions begin in the bowels. According to E. Johansen [Johansen, 2003], current hypotheses connect food allergies with:

– Genetic predisposition
– Dietary factors
– Hyperpermeability of the gut mucosa
– Inflammation of the intestinal epithelium
– Strong bias toward the humoral (antibody-based) type of immunity in newborn infants
– Delay in the development or lack of maturation of the common mucosal immune system, which could be linked to lack of friendly Acidophilus and Bifidobacterium in the gut
– Reactions to parasites and other pathogens invading the system (hygiene hypotheses)

It is much easier to help a child or a teenager with allergies than an adult person. But an adult who is determined to follow a protocol comprising the necessary natural medicine, diet, and cleaning procedures can achieve good results in overcoming allergies.

5.1.2. THE PROCEDURES OF EAV ALLERGY TESTING

Any adverse reaction of the body to substances can be detected by an EAV test. The adverse reaction appears as a higher specific conductivity reading when measured on the skin at the acupuncture meridian points. Allergy testing by EAV has great advantages over other methods such as epicutaneous and intradermal tests, patch tests, challenge (provocation) testing, or avoidance programs. EAV allergy testing is an easy and quick procedure. The time necessary for testing the main allergens, including food and drink, is about one hour.

The method is noninvasive and even suitable for babies. The testing materials (substances) do not enter into direct contact with the bloodstream nor even the skin of the patient. The substance sample is connected with the hand-held electrode. Readings in the range of 40–60 indicate a normal condition. That means that the individual tolerates the substance put into contact with the anode. If the substance irritates the patient, the reading is out of the normal range, usually above 65.

The EAV test is usually done on the point Al-1. This point is sensitive to food allergies. Al-2 can be used for testing some environmental allergens such as inhalants, different types of grass pollens, and chemical substances. It can show the reaction of the lymphatic system to the sample.

Sometimes it is useful to test the effect of a medicine, for example, to see the side effect of the medicine on the liver. In this case, the meridian of the liver is tested without any substance in contact with the anode and after that the same measurement is repeated with the medicine sample in contact with the anode.

Similar tests can be done with vitamins, for example, when we are looking for the best vitamins or supplements to boost the immune system. In this case, the test is carried out against the points of the meridian of the spleen, which is responsible for the reaction of the white and red blood cells involved in cases of inflammation. We are looking for the medicine which when put in contact with the anode is capable of returning the Voll reading in the affected points of the spleen meridian back to a normal condition.

5.1.3. SAMPLE PREPARATION

It is possible to take samples for testing (testers) practically from each state of material: solid, liquid, and gas. The sample can be placed in a container of glass, plastic, or paper. Only a metal container is not suitable. The preparation of the samples includes taking a little piece of the material, putting it in a glass bottle, and if necessary adding 1–2 ml of 90% medical alcohol (Ethanol). The bottle, well-plugged and labeled, can be used for a long time. Dried materials, such as seeds, beans, sugar, or tea do not need alcohol.

It is convenient to divide the testers into groups: proteins, carbohydrates, fruits and vegetables, drinks, chemicals, baby foods, grasses and pollens, animal hairs, and so on.

It is not necessary to prepare samples when working with the Voll machine produced by the BioMeridian company (US), for it has many different allergens included in its computer program repository already. The Russian Ellis machine repository has mostly environmental type allergens, and so all food samples have to be prepared by the Voll method practitioner.

5.1.4. TESTING BABIES AND LITTLE CHILDREN

Children under the age of three years cannot be tested directly. It is said that their meridians are not developed enough to show the energy in a correct way. In addition, their fingers are not big enough for testing. When testing young children less than three years of age, the assistance of a healthy adult person is needed. The adult person's meridians are first tested. Only if these readings are normal is the testing then repeated on the adult again who this time is holding the electrode in contact with the skin of the child. This is convenient and avoids fear and crying in the child. The child can sit comfortably in the lap of his parent and can play with a toy. The child is not allowed to eat during the test.

Allergy testing is useful in supporting the treatment of physical and even emotional disorders. The elimination of some foods from the diet gives the immune and the digestive systems a chance to rest from chronic irritations. Very often, mental and emotional conditions are beneficially affected by changing the diet. For example, children with mental concentration problems improve dramatically when sugar intake is stopped. Women with severe premenstrual syndrome see improvements in their symptoms with a diet of no sugar or wheat. I believe that food allergy testing is a necessary part of any holistic healing.

5.2. ALLERGY AND INTOLERANCE TO FOOD

It is common for people to have allergies to a few foods, but there are people who have allergic reactions to most foods. It is surprising when one can hardly find a group of good foods for them. In general, this shows that their immune system has low energy and that it is irritated. To avoid surprises like this, it is better to start the EAV test first with the immune system (AL) and then with the lymphatic system (Ly). The first four points of the meridian Al can give us a lot of information:

- If only Al-1 is high, it is possible that the problem is in the intestines, so test first for a yeast infection and Candida, and after that for bacterial pathogens.

- If the high signals are only on the right side, it could be a liver, gallbladder, or pancreatic problem.

116

- If the high signals are only on the left side, the problem could be connected with the spleen, so think about viruses, or other intracellular pathogens.

- If the first three points are high, especially Al-3/Al-1a, do a test for parasites.

- If a great many foods appear to be allergens, the most common reason is an invasion by some pathogenic microorganism. Test for bacterial infection.

- If the allergic foods are from one group (carbohydrates, for example), make sure that there is no problem with pancreatic enzymes (test the pancreas, RP/SP, right side), or some pathogen feeding on specific foods. Many bacteria, for example, ferment carbohydrates.

- After that, we test the other organs of the digestive system: intestines (GI/LI, IG/SI), gallbladder (VB/GB), liver (F/LV), stomach (E/ST), and spleen (RP/SP, left side).

- The spleen will reveal if a pathogen is involved.

- If the pancreas is affected, the allergy test does not show real allergy, but intolerance to foods. It is important to remember the meaning of the points of the meridian of the pancreas: RP-1/SP-1 shows protein indigestion, RP-3/SP-1b and RP-5/SP-3 show a carbohydrates problem, RP-4/SP-2 shows uric acid diathesis, RP-5/SP-3 shows indigestion of fatty foods.

Intolerance to food can be caused by an enzyme problem; or by pathogen-producing, system-disturbing toxins. The next step is to detect the pathogen irritating the meridians. The increasing number of scientific articles published in the last thirty-five years state that the intestinal bacterial toxins appear to be injuring the microvilli of the intestinal absorptive cells and the intestinal cell membranes, and as a result causing a variety of inflammatory bowel diseases, including celiac disease, soy protein intolerance, cow's milk intolerance, chronic diarrhea, Crohn's disease, and other disorders [Gotschall, 2003; Gracey, 1981].

In 1991, Dr. J. O. Hunter stated that some food intolerances are not real allergic reactions, but a disorder caused by bacterial fermentation in the intestines. He called this disorder "enterometabolic," or intestinal disorder [Hunter, 1991]. The presence of undigested carbohydrates in the intestines spurs overgrowth of bacteria. Bacterial fermentation occurs, and as a result an excess amount of short-chain organic fatty acids (such as D-lactic acid) are produced and different toxins enter the bloodstream. The problems resulting from bacterial fermentation are connected with acidification of the blood (lower pH) and toxicity, affecting many organs, even the function of the brain [Diez-Gonzalez, Calloway, Kizoulis, & Russell, 1998; Stolberg, Rolfe, Gitlin, Merritt, Mam, Linderer, & Finegold, 1982; Thurn, Pierpont, Ludvigsen, & Eckfeldt, 1985].

The response to an endotoxin of intestinal bacteria is considered an innate immune response, a form of defense mechanism of the immune system. It could stimulate the production of antibodies and cytokines, initiators of an inflammatory process, part of an adaptive immune response [Medzhitov & Janeway, 2000]. Decreasing the amount of fermentable carbohydrates upon which bacteria feed is a reasonable step for improving the immune system.

The other approach, often taken by conventional medicine, is treatment with antibiotics to reduce the population of intestinal bacteria.

The rest of this chapter presents the most common pathogens a Voll practitioner could encounter. The homeopathic and natural medicines identified by EAV tests as effective against these pathogens are mentioned. They work to balance the meridians and to support the immune defense of the human body.

5.3. EAV TESTING FOR DIFFERENT PATHOGENS

The discovery of the main pathogen disturbing the organs, and the immune, lymphatic, and digestive systems of man is a great advantage. Once we know what the pathogen is, we can easily find the necessary way to rebalance the meridian system with a combination of vitamins, supplements, homeopathic remedies, and diet.

First, we must know what pathogens to expect. We should have some knowledge of the most common pathogenic parasites, bacteria, viruses, and fungi. The more we know, the more efficient we become.

That which looks like an art, in fact is based on knowledge, practice, and reading, and following the most advanced frontiers of science. The field of the science of human health should not be divided into small pieces: "This is for general medicine, that is the field of homeopathy, this is technique and computers, here is the field of diets, and this is the field of Chinese medicine. Do not step on the lands of the herbs and do not touch the area of minerals, or do not think about chemical conditions such as pH, red-oxy potential, ion concentration, or the concentration of other substances, this is too much chemistry!" Dividing science into small pieces is not the way to do our work as healers! Only the integration of knowledge can give us a holistic picture and the solutions necessary for solving difficult human health problems. We should realize that regardless of our education and our scientific degrees we know little compared with what is available to be learned. Modestly but persistently we should try our best to learn more and more and to be a little more efficient every day.

The following pages will be an introduction to the field of the microbiology of some species commonly harbored by our bodies and often disturbing our biological systems. The different groups of pathogens have different spectral areas of energy. According to H. Clark [Clark, 1995], the approximate energy bandwidths of families of organisms are as follows:

Tape worms	430–500 KHz
Protozoa, round worms, flat worms	350–450 KHz
Bacteria, Viruses	300–430 KHz
Molds, Fungi	100–350 KHz

Every pathogen has a specific resonance vibration. Pathogen presence in the system indicates that the system energy is weak in the pathogen-specific spectral area. The main point to remember is that the pathogen enters only if the door is open. The second important point is that a pathogen signal does not mean that the disease has already started. The pathogen can be kept under control for a long time, sometimes months, or even years. It is important to support the immune system with specific quantum energy from homeopathic remedies, vitamins, and minerals, to restore the good bacterial flora in the body, to balance the acidity (pH) and red-oxy potential of the system, and to introduce a proper diet. All these help the immune system to restore its energy, to rebalance the meridians, and to eliminate the pathogen. Knowing the pathogens well is helpful for finding the correct technique for their elimination.

5.3.1. EAV DETECTION OF PARASITES

Parasitic infestation is an underestimated medical problem at present. The diagnosis of parasites is possible with blood tests, or stool samples, but very often the parasites are missed and the patients are treated for the wrong disease. Many cases labeled with serious diagnoses such as irritable bowel syndrome, cysts, gallbladder inflammation, endometriosis, asthma, or eczema can be caused by parasites. There are more than five hundred parasites pathogenic to man. They can be classified into three groups:
- Protozoa and Sporozoa are microscopic, single-cell parasites
- Trematodes are flukes and tape worms
- Nematodes are round worms

EAV testing for parasites

Our experience shows that the point Al-3/Al-1a is useful for a quick and accurate EAV test for parasites. The signal from this point is above normal in the case of parasitic infestation. It can be active only on one side of the body in the case of a single parasite like a fluke or cyst in one part of the body. Signals from both sides appear usually when parasites are present in the intestines.

The point Al-3/Al-1a is useful for detecting parasites of any type, large ones, such as Taeniae, small ones such as Oxyuris, or for microscopic Protozoa and Sporozoa such as Amoeba and Toxoplasma.

The point Al-3/Al-1a can be stimulated not only by parasitic infestation, but also by viruses, bacteria, or fungi. Testing for them is essential.

Points Al-1, Al-2, Al-3/Al-1a, and Al-4/Al-1b can be involved and active on both sides of the body in the case of a massive infestation with parasites. The test is positive for the different stages of the parasites: eggs, larvae, cysts, and adults while they are alive. The signal from the point Al-3/Al-1a disappears when the parasites are dead. However, until the remains of the dead parasite are cleared from the organ, a signal for the irritation of the affected organ, not a signal for the parasite, will be present.

The testing for parasites is as follows:
1. Test the point Al-3/Al-1a on both left and right sides; (if the signal is above normal, it could be parasites).

2. Test the same point with antiparasitic medicine, for example Paragon tincture; if the medicine returns the signal to normal, it means that there are parasites in the system.
3. Using specific samples – nosodes for parasites – test for different types of parasites.
4. When the type of parasite has been determined, start testing for the best treatment for this parasite.
5. The best remedy is confirmed only after testing with it in AL-3/Al-1a returns the signal to normal.

Very good results for parasites are achieved with herbal medicines such as PARA-90 and Paragon tincture. The latter is useful for children, because the dose can be easily counted: from 3 drops in fruit juice for babies above 6 months old to 20 drops in water for adults twice a day.

Usually, the treatment with medication for parasites lasts for one month.

The Zapper machine (vibration with frequency 33 KHz, which is the general vibration for parasites) of Dr. H. Clark works very well, too. The specific resonance frequencies of the parasites, given in her book [Clark, 1995] work well. The Driver Resonator machine, produced in South Africa, is used successfully for body detoxification and cleansing of different pathogens. Table 7 (in the Appendix) shows homeopathic remedies that are good for treating parasites. Their action is confirmed by Voll testing.

5.3.1.1. PROTOZOA AND SPOROZOA

These are microscopic parasites affecting the blood and other organs. The most common parasites from this group are:

– **Amoeba (Entamoeba histolytica, Entamoeba coli, Naegleria)** affect the gut lumen and cause diarrhea and vomiting; the liver, gallbladder, lungs, and brain can also be affected.

The resonance vibrations of 397–400.35 KHz and 381.1–387.8 KHz are useful for eliminating these parasites [Clark, 1995].

Homeopathic medicine for Amoeba
We obtained the best results treating an amoebic invasion when using Paragon herbal drops in combination with the homeopathic remedies

121

Acidum aceticum, Acidum phosphoricum, Bryonia, and Carbo Vegetabilis. Another effective homeopathic remedy for Amoeba, according to EAV tests by Usupov, is Aloe [Usupov, 2000]. Oxygen-producing Cellfood drops work well for Amoeba, too (Table 7).

Other Protozoa and Sporozoa are:

- **Babesia microti** and **Babesia divergens** are haemoprotozoan parasites causing symptoms similar to those of malaria. Their host can be a little tick, which can help them invade animals and man. Our EAV tests confirmed the effective action of the homeopathic remedies China and Cuprum metallicum against Babesia protozoa. The herbal tincture Paragon works well, too (Table 7).

- **Balantidium Coli** causes diarrhea and weight loss.

- **Ciliates (Subphylum ciliophora)** in the gut lumen and tissues cause bloody dysentery.

- **Giardia intestinalis (Lamblia intestinalis)** affects the mucosa of the intestines.

Homeopathic remedies for Giardia (Lamblia)
A good homeopathic remedy for Giardiasis, confirmed with EAV tests by G. A. Usupov [Usupov, 2000], is Berberis. We use Zincum picricum with good results (Table 7).

- **Leishmania donovani** causes progressive damage of the liver and spleen, dysentery, and bleeding of the mucous membranes.

- Malaria is caused by a blood parasite of the genus **Plasmodium (Pl. falciparum, Pl. vivax, Pl. ovale, Pl. malariae)**. There are more than 156 species that invade the deep tissues and cause serious damage to the liver and spleen.

For all of them the herbal tincture Paragon works well. An individual homeopathic medicine is recommended after EAV testing.

Homeopathic medicine for Malaria
The homeopathic remedies for Malaria according to the R. Murphy

Repertory [Murphy, 1996:423] are: Abies nigra, Argentum nitricum, Arnica, Bryonia, Carbolicum acidum, Cedron, China, Chininum arsenicosum, Chininum sulphuricum, Eucaliyptus, Eupatorium perfoliatum, Ferrum metallicum, Ipeca, Lycopodium, Natrium muriaticum, Natrium sulphuricum, Nux vomica, Opium, Psorinum, Sulphur, Terebinthina, and Veratrum viride.

Homeopathic medicine for Malaria confirmed by Voll testing

The remedies with the best results for Malaria confirmed by our Voll testing are: Borax, China, Chininum arsenicosum, Chininum sulphuricum, Carbo vegetabilis, Lachesis, Malaria nosode, and Nux vomica (Table 7).

– **Toxoplasma** (from the group sporozoa) invades the cells of the gut epithelium, lungs, muscles, and CNS, and it can cause toxoplasma encephalitis. In some cases Toxoplasma can cause endometriosis and infertility.

Homeopathic medicine for Toxoplasma

The best results for treating Toxoplasma we obtained by using the homeopathic remedy Cina. Usupov [Usupov, 2000] using EAV tests found the most successful remedy to be Zincum picricum (Table 7). The herbal tincture Paragon works very well.

– **Trichomonas group** – **Tr. tenax** in the mouth; **Tr. hominis** in the bowels in the area of the caecum; and **Tr. Vaginalis**, which causes urethritis and vaginal inflammation with a yellow-green discharge.

Homeopathic medicine for Trichomonas

According to Usupov [Usupov, 2000], good results treating Trichomonas are obtained with the homeopathic remedies Helonias and Clematis (Table 7).

– **Trypanosoma** – **T. cruzi** causes Chagas disease in America; **T. brucei gambiense** causes a disease similar to that known as Sleeping sickness in Africa with pyrexia, edema of the face, meningitis, encephalitis, and heart damage.

Homeopathic remedies for Sleeping sickness

The following homeopathic remedies are listed for Sleeping sickness

123

in R. Murphy's Repertory [Murphy, 1996:439]: Arsenicum album, Gelsemium, Nux moshata, and Opium.

5.3.1.2. TREMATODES

This group of parasites includes flukes and tape worms of which there are many different types. The most common are as follows:

- **Bilharzia (Schistosomiasis)** caused by blood trematodes of the genus **Schistosoma mansoni, S. haematobium, S. japonicum, and S. intercalatum.** The blood stage of the worm can invade many different organs, mainly the veins, bowels, liver, spleen, and bladder. Mimicry of the blood stage of the Schistosome worm is registered, which covers its surface in molecules picked up from the blood of its host and lives completely camouflaged, hidden from the immune system. It sometimes makes the laboratory test for this type of worm inconclusive [Playfair, 2004].

The frequencies used for helping the immune system in a Bilharzia invasion are 473 and 353 KHz [Clark, 1995].

Homeopathic medicine for Bilharzia
The homeopathic medicines given for Bilharzia in R. Murphy's Repertory [Murphy, 1996] are: Antimonium tartaricum, Arsenicum album, and China [Murphy, 1996].

Homeopathic medicine for Bilharzia, confirmed by the Voll test
We obtained the best results after EAV testing for Bilharzia when we used Antimonium tartaricum, Zincum metallicum, Zincum picricum, and Zincum valerianicum. Usupov [Usupov, 2000] shows that the remedy Secale cornutum is effective against Bilharzia, too (Table 7).

- **Diphyllobothrium latum** is a fish tape worm which can be caught from eating raw fish. It lives in the small intestines and can reach a size of 10 m.

- **Echinococcus granulosus** causes Hydatid disease, where big hydatid cysts are formed in the liver, lungs, brain, and other organs.

Homeopathic medicine for Echinococcus

By EAV tests Usupov [Usupov, 2000] confirmed the action of the homeopathic remedies Apis and Hydrastis for Echinococcus (Table 7).

- **Fasciola hepatica** (sheep liver fluke) invades the duodenum, liver, and bile ducts.

- **Fasciolopsis buski** is the largest intestinal fluke in man. It can reach 75 mm in length. Usually found in the bowels, it can also be located in other organs including the liver, the gallbladder, the pancreas, and the kidneys. It can be found also in the ovaries and uterus in different stages of its life cycle and it can cause thickening and inflammation of the endometrium, known as Endometriosis.

- **Opisthorchis viverrini** is Southeast Asian liver fluke.

- **O. felineus** is Cat liver fluke.

- **Paragonimus westmani** is known as Lung fluke, but can also be found in the duodenum, brain, heart, spinal cord, and muscles.

- *Taenia saginata* is Bovine tape worm.

- **Taenia solum** is Swine tape worm.

- **Taenia pisiformis** is Canine tape worm.

Homeopathic remedies for Taenia

The homeopathic remedies for Taenia are: Ailanthus glandulosa, Calcarea carbonica, Carbo animalis, Carbo vegetabilis, Filix-mas, Formica rufa, Granatum, Graphites, Natrium carbonicum, Platina, Pulsatilla, Sabadilla, Sepia, Silica, and Stannum [Murphy, 1996].

When treating parasites it is generally best to first prescribe herbal preparations and then to test the affected organs for the homeopathic remedies and the natural supplements that would provide the organs with the best support.

125

5.3.1.3. NEMATODES

Nematode is the Latin name for round worms. It is difficult to describe even a small number of the multitude of these parasites.

- **Ascaris lumbricoides** is the most common one in humans. They live in the bowels and can grow to a size of up to 35 cm. They cause digestive disorders. Part of their life cycle is the migration of the larvae to the lungs where they cause coughing when lying in bed. Children who have Ascaris are anxious at night. They have stomach and abdominal discomfort after meals, and even after drinks. A rash often appears on the stomach and on the chest. Many cases of eczema can be caused by the presence of Ascaris worms.

Many people live with Ascaris infestation without serious complaints for a long time. Our practice, however, shows that these types of worms are accompanied by bacterial infection in the bowels, very often Clostridium difficile, and this finding confirms the work of Dr. H. Clarke [Clark, 1995].

Homeopathic remedies for Ascaris worms
The main homeopathic remedies for Ascaris worms in R. Murphy's Repertory [Murphy, 1996:385] (given under Ascarides) are: Arsenicum album, Baryta carbonica, Calcarea carbonica, Chelonias, Cina, Ferrum metallicum, Ignatia, Magnesium sulphuricum, Natrium muriaticum, Natrium phosphoricum, Ptelea trifoliata, Ratanhia peruviana, Sabadilla, Santalum album, Scirrhinum, Sepia, Silica, Sinapis nigra, Spigelia, Spongia, Sulphur, Terebinthina, Teucrium, and Valeriana.
According to Usupov [Usupov, 2000], the remedy Cina was confirmed by the Voll test (Table 7).

- **Ancylostoma (Hookworm)** is the second most common human helminthic infection after Ascaris. It penetrates the skin and reaches the small intestine.

Homeopathic remedies for Hookworm
The homeopathic remedies for Hookworm are: Carduus marianus, Chenopodium anthelminticum, and Thymol [Murphy, 1996].

126

- **Trichuris triura (whipworm)** is the third most common nematode, reaching a size of 4 cm and living in the small intestine in the area of the caecum.

- **Enterobius vermicularis (Oxyuris, Pin worms)** are small nematodes, common in young children. They cause loss of weight, itchy anus, and anxiety at night.

Homeopathic remedies for Pin worms

The homeopathic remedies for Pin worms listed in R. Murphy's Repertory under Oxyuris vermicularis [Murphy, 1996:429] are: Arsenicum album, Baptisia, Helonias, Cina, Ignatia, Indigo, Lycopodium, Mercurius dulcis, Mercurius solubilis, Natrium phosphoricum, Ratanhia, Santoninum, Silica, Sinapis nigra, Spigelia, Teucrium, and Valeriana. Usupov had confirmed, by EAV tests, the beneficial action of Cina and Carbo animalis for Pin worm cases [Usupov, 2000]. Our experience shows that Spigelia and Calcarea carbonica are very good, too (Table 7).

- **Mansonella perstans and M. ozzardi** are nematodes that cause the sickness Loa loa, which invades subcutaneous tissue, spinal fluid, the urinary system, the lungs, and peripheral blood.

- **Strongyloides stercoralis** invades the lungs, stomach, and intestine.

- **Trichinella spiralis** invades the intestine and causes diarrhea and nausea. The larva can settle in the muscles and this may cause muscle pain.

Homeopathic medicine for Trichinella spiralis

A good homeopathic remedy for Trichinella spiralis, confirmed by Usupov [Usupov, 2000] with EAV tests, is Secale cornutum (Table 7).

- **Wuchereria bancrofti** causes Filariasis. The worm invades the lymphatic vessels and lymph nodes.

The main homeopathic remedies for worms

The main remedies for worms, given in R. Murphy's Repertory [Murphy, 1996:449], are: Ambrosia artemisiae, Arsenicum album, Calcarea carbonica, Carcinosinum, Chelonias, Cicuta virosa, Cina, Ferrum metallicum, Ferrum muriaticum, Gaertner, Granatum, Naphthalinum, Natrium muriaticum, Natrium phosphoricum, Nux moshata, Ratanhia, Ruta, Sabadilla, Santalum album, Silica, Sinapis nigra, Spigelia, Stannum, Sulphur, Terebinthina, Valeriana, Viola odorata, and Viola tricolor.

5.3.2. EAV AND HOMEOPATHY FOR BACTERIAL PATHOGENS

5.3.2.1. CLOSTRIDIUM

Clostridium is a broad genus of Gram-positive (some are Gram-negative) spore-bearing bacteria growing in soil, in water, and in decomposing plant and animal matter. Some species are anaerobic by nature, some are aerobic. They need a low red-oxy potential medium in order to sporulate and to grow. If the oxygen is increased, it inhibits their multiplication [Mackie & McCartney, 1978]. It is important to note that in the case of Clostridium, any antioxidants (substances giving electrons) aggravate the infection, and the intake of oxidants (substances accepting electrons) helps fight the infection. During our practice, we discovered that the healing process of anaerobic bacteria requires stopping the intake of Vitamins A, C, and E, and other antioxidants. On the hand, Cellfood drops and magnesium peroxide powder, releasing oxygen, are useful. One characteristic property of Clostridium bacteria is pleomorphism, that is, they can exist in different shapes depending on the conditions of the milieu: rods, rods with filaments, citron bodies, spindle- or club-shaped; and they can change from Gram-positive to Gram-negative. It would be interesting to use dark field microscopy to research the presence of bacterial rods in the live blood of patients before and after Voll testing, followed by the appropriate homeopathic treatments. Such research could be a bridge among the three fields of natural medicine: Enderlein's theory [Enderlein, 1916], homeopathy, and the EAV method of Dr. Voll.

There are many pathogenic species of the Clostridium genus. Among them are Cl. welchii (Cl. perfringens) and Cl. sporogenes, which are both part of the normal flora of the gut of man. The bacteria occur in the large intestine of healthy man. Abnormal growth can start in the small intestines, producing many types of toxins, some of them lethal and necrotizing.

Clostridium difficile is another species affecting the digestive system of man. It causes bowel infections. The most common symptoms are diarrhea with cramps and abdominal pain, acute and chronic. In heavy infections it can cause membranous colitis. Research group reports indicate that Clostridium difficile is likely to have been responsible for the increased hospitalization and death rates from enteric bacterial pathogens in the US during the period 1992–1998. The results show that Clostridium difficile is the first invader among the five types of bacteria causing heavy diarrhea: Clostridium difficile, Yersinia enterocolitica, Campylobacter, Pseudomonas, and Staphylococcus [Frost, Cann, & Calderon, 1998].

Other pathogenic species from the Clostridium genus are: Cl. acetobutylicum, Cl. septicum, Cl. oedematiens (Cl. novyi), Cl. tetani, Cl. botulinum, Cl. bifermentans, Cl. sordellii, and Cl. hystolyticum. Each has its own subspecies and pleomorphic forms. They are very toxic, causing gas gangrene, tetanus, food poisoning, and blood poisoning.

The species of Clostridium bacteria are more sugar-transforming, i.e. saccharolytic, and less protein-transforming. This means that the most important step for a diet supporting the immune system of individuals with Clostridium infection is eliminating the intake of sugar. We found this to be the best diet and necessary during the period of the treatment for Clostridium. The main features of the diet are: no sugar, but fructose is allowed; no wheat, but rye is allowed; no milk and cheese, but yogurt and butter are allowed (Table 4).

The research of Dr. H. Clark [Clark, 1995] shows resonance frequencies for Clostridium in the spectral areas: 361.0–364.55 KHz; 362.05–365.6 KHz; 382.8–391.15 KHz; 394.2–398.1 KHz.

Homeopathic remedies for Clostridium difficile infections

The homeopathic remedies for Clostridium infections given in the Repertory of R. Murphy [Murphy, 1996] are as follows:

p. 410, Gangrene: Agaricus, Anthracinum, Arsenicum album, Asafoetida, Belladonna, Cantharis, Carbo animalis, Carbo vegetabilis, Causticum, China, Colchicum, Crotalus horridus, Iodum, Kalium phosphoricus, Kreosotum, Lachesis, Phosphorus, Plumbum metallicum, Rhus toxicodendron, Sabina, Secale, Silicea, and Stramonium.

129

p. 442, Tetanus: Aconitum, Angustura vera, Argentum nitricum, Belladonna, Calendula, Camphorum, Cantharis, Causticum, Cedron, Cicuta, Cocculus, Croton, Cuprum metallicum, Cuprum aceticum, Gelsemium, Glonoinum, Hepar sulphur, Hyoscyamus, Hypericum, Ipecacuanha, Laurocerasus, Ledum, Lycopodium, Mercurius, Moschus, Nux moscata, Nux vomica, Oenanthe, Opium, Passiflora, Plantago, Platinum metallicum, Plumbum metallicum, Secale, Stramonium, and Strychninum.

Homeopathic remedies for Clostridium difficile confirmed by Voll test

Using the Voll machine for testing Clostridium difficile in the digestive tract, we found that the following homeopathic remedies work very well: Acidum carbolicum, Acidum nitricum, Acidum floricum, Acidum phosphoricum, Acidum picricum, Acidum sarcolacticum, Acidum sulphuricum, Argentum nitricum, Arsenicum iodatum, Arsenicum sulphuricum flavum, Bismuthum metallicum, Borax, Bryonia album, Ceanothus americanus, Chelidonius, Cuprum metallicum, Gelsemium, Hepar sulphuris, Kalium bichromicum, Kalium iodatum, Mercurius corrosivus, Nux vomica, and Secale cornutum (Table 3).

EAV testing for Clostridium difficile

Our research was carried out on Clostridium difficile affecting the digestive tract of man. The patients usually have pain in the abdomen, cramping, bloated abdomen full of gas, and often diarrhea with a bad smell. They complain of a metal taste and bad breath in the mouth. The presence of this bacterium manifests itself first at the point Al-1 (immune system, right side). The meridians of the colon (GI/LI) and small intestines (IG/SI) have to be tested, too. More often the signals for irritation come from the right side. Cl. difficile is detected often on points IG-1/SI-1 (ileum and appendix) and IG-2/SI-2 (lymphatic vessels of the duodenum). The bacterium can cause inflammation in the gallbladder, so it is essential to test the meridian VB/GB. In cases of Cl. difficile in the digestive system, it is often the liver that is affected (especially F-1/LV-1); also the gallbladder (VB/GB), the pancreas (RP/SP), and the kidneys (R/KI). In many cases with chronic high cholesterol proved by blood tests and controlled by medications, the cholesterol level is lowered after clearing Cl. difficile from the bowels.

130

Many cases with cholecystitis and gallstones were detected with signals for Cl. difficile in the gallbladder.

This bacterium causes severe headaches with chronic redness of the eyes. The headaches are often worse in the morning, or especially after taking a glass of wine or chocolate. Key symptoms for diagnosing Cl. difficile are the craving for chocolate and strong aggravation after drinking wine, combined with chronic redness of the sclera. Many cases of acne in teenagers are greatly improved after cleaning the system of Cl. difficile. Good results for reducing Cl. difficile in the bowel are achieved by using a combination of one of the homeopathic remedies listed above and the homeopathic nosode for the bacterium. Adding a resonance vibration 365 KHz and increasing the level of oxygen in the blood by taking Cellfood oxygen drops or magnesium peroxide powder support the treatment.

The treatment needs three to four months and has to be supported by a proper diet (Table 4).

5.3.2.2. YERSINIA

The bacteria in the genus Yersinia are known as well as Pasteurella and Francisella. They are small, oval, Gram-negative bacilli, extremely polymorphic, changing their size and shape under certain conditions. They can be aerobic or anaerobic, but are sensitive to oxygen therapy.

- **Yersinia pestis** is the cause of bubonic plague and pneumonic plague, responsible for the most terrible epidemic periods in the history of Europe. The source of the infection for man is in black rats.

- **Yersinia pseudotuberculosis** causes heavy infections of the lungs, liver, spleen, and mesenteric lymph nodes, and can cause erythema nodosum. The infection comes from rats.

- **Pasteurella multocida (Pasteurella septica)** can cause hemorrhagic septicemia in animals and birds. In man it can cause local abscesses after an animal bite, meningitis after a head injury, and respiratory infections.

- **Francisella tularensis** causes disease in rodents and rabbits and can be transmitted to man by flies or by direct contact with infected

131

animals or contaminated water. The condition is named Tularemia and it includes typhoid fever characterized by an ulcer at the site of infection, and inflamed and ulcerating lymph nodes.

Yersinia enterocolitica is one of the five enteric bacterial pathogens in present times causing serious cases of diarrhea, ending with hospitalization [Frost, Cann, & Calderon, 1998]. The infection is expressed as severe diarrhea, acute ileitis, mesenteric adenitis, appendicitis, and erythema nodosum. The resonance frequencies found from practice to be useful for Yersinia enterocolitica are: 184 KHz, 353 KHz, and 378 KHz.

The Voll test in cases of Yersinia enterocolitica show that the foods dairy products, sugar, and fructose should be excluded from the menu (Table 4).

EAV testing for Yersinia bacteria

The Voll test includes immune system (AL left and right), lymphatic system (Ly, MC-8/CI-8), intestines (GI/LI, IG/SI), liver (F/LV), gallbladder (VB/GB), and spleen (RP/SP, left).

Homeopathic remedies for Yersinia bacteria

The main remedies for Yersinia found in the R. Murphy Repertory [Murphy, 1996] are: p. 390, under Bubonic plague: Arsenicum album, Baptisia, Bufo rana, Carbo animalis, Carcinosinum, Cinnabaris, Hepar sulphuris, Hippozaeninum, Kalium iodatum, Lachesis, Mercurius solubilis, Nitricum acidum, Silica; under Burning bubo: Carbo animalis, Tarentula cubensis; under Suppurating bubo: Aurum metallicum, Carbo animalis, Hepar sulphuris, Iodum, Kalium iodatum, Lachesis, Mercurius solubilis, Mercurius iodatus ruber, Silica, and Sulphur.

Homeopathic remedies for Yersinia enterocolitica, confirmed by Voll testing

Our research using EAV tests showed that the following remedies normalize the signal from the bacterium Yersinia enterocolitica: Arsenicum iodatum, Bismuthum metallicum, Bismuthum subnitricum, Bufo rana, Calcarea iodata, China, Cinnabaris, Hepar sulphur, Hydrastis, Kalium bichromicum, Magnesium muriaticum, Thuja, and Veratrum album.

Usupov [Usupov, 2000] confirmed the action of the remedy Kreosotum (Table 3).

The diet is an important part of the treatment (Table 4). In chronic cases the medications and the diet should continue for three months. Increased oxygen in the digestive system and treatment with resonance vibration are beneficial, too.

5.3.2.3. RICKETTSIA

The Rickettsia are a large family of primitive prokaryotic cells, with obligate intracellular existence. They live and multiply in the cytoplasm of the cells. Their size of 200–500 nm is small in comparison with bacteria but larger than viruses. Their shape and form is polymorphic and changable: rod-shaped, oval, or sometimes filamentous. The different types of Rickettsia find hosts among lice, fleas, ticks, mites, birds, and mammals. The infection can be transmitted to man through insect bite, milk, meat, inhalation of insects' feces, or infection agents rubbed into the skin.

Epidemic forms of Rickettsia have been known in the past as typhus, spotted fever, scrub typhus, French fever, Q-fever, and many others. These infections were responsible for heavy and excruciating illnesses causing millions of deaths. Nowadays, there are slowly evolving, less-virulent forms, which are nevertheless able to induce long-lasting vascular and neurological pathologies.

The discovery and investigations of these pathogens was done by a number of brave and self-denying scientists: H. T. Ricketts (1909), S. von Prowazek, Ch. Nicolle, P. Giroid, Professor J. B. Jadin, and recently C. L. Jadin, while she was working in South Africa [Jadin, 1999; Mackie & McCartney, 1978; Jadin, 2002].

There are many pathogens causing Rickettsia group maladies. Among them the most commonly known are: R. prowazekii—typhus (from lice, rats), R. rickettsii—Rocky mountain spotted fever (from ticks), R. mooseri or R. typhi—typhus (from fleas), R. sibirica—Siberian typhus (from ticks), R. acari—fever (from mites), R. australis—fever (from ticks), R. tsutsugamushi—typhus (from mites), R. quintana—French fever (lice), and Coxiella burnetti—Q fever (ticks).

From the entry point in the skin, lungs, and digestive mucosa, the infection spreads via the bloodstream to infect the vascular endothelium.

133

The microorganisms grow and multiply in the cytoplasm of the cells until their number becomes so great that the cells burst and a multitude of them are released into the bloodstream. While the Rickettsia are in the cytoplasm of the cells, this is the asymptomatic stage of the infection; after they are released the host will display various symptoms and this is the origin of the diseases such as:

- Chronic Fatigue Syndrome,
- Fibromyalgia,
- Cardiovascular diseases of the blood vessels and heart valves,
- Neurological diseases such as meningoencephalitis,
- Abdominal diseases such as appendicitis, gallbladder, and liver problems,
- Ocular diseases such as uveitis, retinal angiopathy, optic neuritis,
- Autoimmune diseases such as rheumatoid and psoriatic arthritis, lupus, and others [Mackie & McCartney; Frost, Cann, & Calderon, 1998; Jadin, 2002].

Because the infection can happen in any organ, the Rickettsia symptom spectrum is wide: tiredness, sleepiness, headaches, muscular and arthritic pain, loss of balance, vision abnormalities, Raynaud's syndrome, nausea, recurrent sore throat, memory and concentration problems, chest pain and palpitations, low-grade fever, bruising, neurological and psychological disorders [Jadin, 2002].

The special Microagglutination test of Giroid–Jadin detects the three main strains of Rickettsia (R. prowazekii, R. mooseri, R. conorii), Coxiella burnetti, and Neorickettsia Chlamydia Q18. Traditional Rickettsial infection treatments last long and follow special protocols for the administration of antibiotics from the tetracycline group. A problem with this treatment is recurrent symptoms and infection tendency, caused by the pathogen's ability to hide for a long time in the cells, appearing undetectable and unapproachable by the body's immune defense system.

Finding successful Rickettsial treatments is a huge challenge for medical professionals and of great importance to millions of people. That is why a test, with the potential of EAV, and a mild, nontoxic treatment such as homeopathic medicine, deserve attention and further research, which will hopefully include specialists in this medical field.

EAV testing for Rickettsia

The test depends on the samples (testers) available. The more nosodes for different species of Rickettsia are combined in the sample, the better results can be obtained for detecting the pathogens. It is essential to test the pancreas and spleen (RP/SP), immune and lymphatic systems (AI, Ly), liver (F/LV), kidneys and bladder (R/KI and V/UB), intestines (GI/LI; IG/SI), lungs (P/LU), meridian of joints (Ad/JO), nerves (Nd/NE), and if necessary other meridians, according to the sufferer's complaints.

The Rickettsial infections treatment has to be in the form of a combination of remedies, diet, and vibration and seriously followed for three to six months. It is necessary to test the remedy on the meridian of the spleen, and after that, if it works, it should be tested on the meridians of the other affected organs. Our research in resonance vibrations showed that the following vibrational frequencies are useful for supporting the immune system in cases of Rickettsial infection: 10.8 Hz, 1,080 Hz, 10.8 KHz, 33 KHz, 128 KHz, 325KHz, 361 KHz. The most useful resonance vibrations are underlined. The diet for Rickettsia cases excludes dairy, sugar, wheat, alcohol, and soy products (Table 4). It is also important to test the spleen meridian points for oxidants and antioxidants that adjust the red-oxy potential of the system of each individual. Oxygen and Vitamin B-complex are usually beneficial.

Homeopathic remedies for Rickettsial pathogens

The main remedies for Rickettsia can be found in the Repertory of R. Murphy [Murphy, 1996:446]: Typhoid fever—Acidum aceticum, Acidum fluoricum, Acidum phosphoricum, Acidum sulphuricum, Agaricus, Alumina, Aluminum metallicum, Apis, Apocynum, Arnica, Arsenicum, Arum triphyllum, Asarum europaeum, Atropinum, Baptisia, Baryta carbonica, Belladonna, Berberis, Bryonia alba, Caladium, Calcarea carbonica, Camphora, Cantharis, Capsicum, Carbo animalis, Carbo vegetabilis, Chamomilla, Chelidonium, Chininum arsenicosum, Chininum sulphuricum, China, Chlorinum, Cimicifuga, Cocculus, Colchicum, Crotalus horridus, Echinacea, Eucalyptis, Ferrum metallicum, Gelsemium, Hyoscyamus, Iodum, Lachesis, Laurocerasus, Lycopodium, Magnesium phosphoricus, Mancinella, Mercurius solubilis, Mercurius cyanatus,

135

Moschus, Muriaticum acidum, Nitricum acidum, Nitri spiritus dulcis, Nux moshata, Nux vomica, Opium, Phosphorus, Psorinum, Pyrogenium, Rhus tox, Secale cornutum, Sepia, Silica, Sinapis nigra, Stramonium, Sulphur, Taraxacum, Terebinthina, Urtica urens, Valeriana, Veratrum album, Veratrum viride, and Zincum metallicum.

Homeopathic remedies for Rickettsial pathogens, confirmed by Voll testing

Our Voll testing showed that for Rickettsial infection the best working homeopathic remedies are: Acidum muriaticum, Agaricus, Apis, Arnica, Arsenicum album, Arsenicum iodatum, Arsenicum sulphuricum flavum, Baptisia, Bellis perennis, Bryonia alba, Carbo vegetabilis, Chelidonium, China, Chininum arsenicosum, Colchicum, Crotalus horridus, Ignatia, Lachesis, Mercurius cyanatus, and Veratrum album (Table 3).

5.3.2.4. CHLAMYDIA

The genus Chlamydia consists of primitive cells (prokaryotes) living in the cytoplasm of host cells. They are intracellular parasites, real energy parasites, because they take energy from compounds such as Adenosine Triphosphate (ATP), the molecule which is the carrier of energy to the cells. Chlamydia is capable of synthesizing its own DNA, the molecule carrier of genetic material, from ATP, so it is not a virus, regardless of its small size. There are two polymorphic forms of Chlamydia:

– small, 300 nm, cell with a compact dense nucleoid. This is a very infectious form.

– large, from 800 nm to 1200 nm, cell without a dense nucleoid. It can divide into two and condense to the small form in 24–48 hours.

Chlamydia affects birds, sheep, cattle, goats, pigs, and other animals.

There are two species known to infect man: Chlamydia trachomatis and Chlamydia psittaci. In man, the infection can take two forms:

– Ornitosis or Psittacosis (PLT), which affects the respiratory tract and causes fever and flu-like symptoms, and

– Genital infection with trachoma-inclusion conjunctivitis-lymphogranuloma venereum (TRIS-LGV), with complications, including meningoencephalitis, pneumonia, arthritis, pericarditis, myocarditis, and typhoid state with enlarged liver and spleen

The eyes are often affected, even babies can have Chlamydia infection. It can cause inclusion conjunctivitis-trachoma, or keratitis, causing blindness. Swimming pool conjunctivitis could be caused by Chlamydia too. In man, the infection can cause non-specific urethritis and prostatitis. In women it affects the cervix and the fallopian tubes and it can cause infertility. Chlamydia infection is much more widespread than it is thought, because sometimes there are no clinical symptoms. M. Boiadjiev found that in many homeopathic cases, which did not respond well to a chosen constitutional remedy, the remedy started working after applying the homeopathic nosode for Chlamydia [Boiadjiev, 2000].

According to Dr. H. Clark, the resonance frequency for Chlamydia is in the interval 379.70–383.95 KHz [Clark, 1995].

The food tests in cases of Chlamydia infections show that wheat, vinegar, and alcohol aggravate the disease the most (Table 4).

EAV testing for Chlamydia

The EAV test for Chlamydia needs to be applied on most of the meridians, because the pathogen affects many organs. It is essential to include in the test the meridians of the immune and lymphatic systems (Al, Ly), liver (F/LV), pancreas and spleen (RP/SP), lungs (P/LU), kidneys (R/KI), bowels (GI/LI, IG/SI), and joints (Ad/JO).

Homeopathic remedies for Chlamydia
In the Repertory of R. Murphy, three remedies are given under Chlamydial infection: Medorrhinum, Sulphur, and Thuja [Murphy, 1996].

Homeopathic remedies for Chlamydia, confirmed by Voll testing
Using a Voll machine for testing, we found many remedies working well for Chlamydial infections: Acidum nitricum, Acidum picricum, Argentum nitricum, Aconitum, Aethusa, Agaricus, Arsenicum sulphuricum flavum, Bryonia, Kali iodatum, Kreosotum, Lachesis, Mercurius cyanatum, Mercurius vivus, Pyrogen, Sabina, and Sanicula. Usupov [Usupov, 2000], using the EAV test, confirmed the remedy Rumex (Table 3). Vitamin C,

137

Vitamin B complex, and antioxidants work very well for a Chlamydial infection, too.

5.3.2.5. CAMPYLOBACTER AND HELICOBACTER

Campylobacter is a genus of spiral, motile, Gram-negative bacteria. Species of Campylobacter are a common cause of food poisoning with headache, nausea, diarrhea, and vomiting. The species Campylobacter jejunum is often found in cases with chronic discomfort of the digestive system and a tendency for diarrhea. The species Campylobacter pylori is known as Helicobacter pylori. H. pylori is a bacterium causing chronic and acute gastritis, duodenitis, peptic ulcers, metaplasia, and in some cases cancer of the stomach and duodenum. It is known that more than 90% of cases of duodenal ulcers are caused by H. pylori. There are thirteen species of this genus, similar in their action, and causing lifelong infection in most cases. The medical diagnosis of H. pylori is done by gastroscopy, biopsy, and histological, cytological, and serological tests, or by the Snabb-urease test. Similar symptoms are caused by other bacteria such as Proteus mirabilis and Klebsiella pneumoniae. The antibiotics treatment, combined with acid pump inhibitor, gives good results. Nowadays, however, it has become more problematic due to the increased resistance of the bacteria. Another approach is Bismuth salts treatment, which has been known for centuries. Dr. H. Clark found resonance frequencies for Campylobacter bacteria in the intervals 352.0–357.2 KHz and 365.3–370.6 KHz [Clark, 1995]. Increased oxygen inhibits the bacteria, too. The diet should exclude dairy, sugar, alcohol, and soy products (Table 4).

EAV testing for the bacteria Campylobacter and Helicobacter

The EAV test for Campylobacter and H. pylori is based on measurements of the meridian of the immune system (Al), the stomach meridian (E/ST), and the meridians of the large and small intestines (GI/LI) (IG/SI). The EAV measurements show that the infection can spread to other organs of the digestive system such as the pancreas (RP/SP) and the gallbladder (VB/GB). First, the point Al-1 will show the presence of the bacteria, and after that the most sensitive points are on the meridian of the stomach (E/ST-1 to 8).

Homeopathic remedies for Campylobacter and Helicobacter, confirmed by Voll testing

We found only one remedy, Anacardium, specific to these bacteria, that was described in the literature, by Usupov who confirmed the remedy using Voll testing [Usupov, 2000]. Our own investigations by Voll testing revealed that the best working homeopathic remedies for Campylobacter and Helicobacter are: Alumina, Anacardium, Arsenicum album, Arsenicum iodatum, Bismuthum metallicum, Bismuthum subnitricum, Cadmium metallicum, Hypericum, Phosphorus, Veratrum album, Zincum metallicum, and Zincum Phosphoricum (Table 3).

5.3.2.6. ESCHERICHIA COLI

Escherichia coli (E-coli) is a genus of Gram-negative, big in size (3,000 nm), aerobic, and facultatively anaerobic bacteria of the family Enterobacteriaceae. E-coli builds colonies, fermenting glucose and lactose. The bacterium is part of the normal flora of the human gut [Kiehn, 2002], but it is also associated with diseases. Uropathogenic strains of E-coli may cause 90% of urinary tract infections in humans. Neonatal meningitis caused by E-coli is another serious and dangerous complication for infants. Five types of pathogenic diarrhea causing strains of E-coli are now recognized:

- Enterotoxigenic strains, producing toxins similar to the cholera toxin and resulting in diarrhea without fever.

- Enteroinvasive strains, penetrating within epithelial cells of the colon and causing cell destruction with diarrhea and fever. Enteropathogenic strains, producing enterotoxin, similar to that of Shigella and inducing a watery diarrhea.

- Enteroaggregative strains, producing Hemolysin and Enteroaggregative ST-toxin which cause non-bloody diarrhea.

- Enterohemorrhagic group, especially the strain E-coli 0157:H7, produced by acquiring pieces of DNA of bacterial virus in its genetic code, having properties of a virus and producing a toxin named SLT, or Verotoxin. It causes hemorrhaging from the intestines and Hemolytic Uremic Syndrome (HUS). Both are dangerous to infants up to two years of age.

Very often E-coli causes chronic and difficult urinary tract infections. It can be found causing appendicular abscesses, peritonitis, cholecystitis, wound infections, and other infections. In our practice we saw some prominent E-coli infection cases diagnosed with Insulin resistance. E-coli are one of the most resistant-to-antibiotics bacteria of our time. This is why the Voll test and homeopathy have a place as methods for controlling it. The resonance frequencies of E-coli according to H. Clark [Clark, 1995] are 356 KHz and 392–393 KHz. Increased oxygen inhibits the bacteria. Useful for E-coli urinary infections are herbal teas, such as Bearberry leaves, Berberis, and Sarsaparilla, alkalized by addition of bicarbonate of soda (NaHCO3).

EAV testing for E-coli

The EAV test for E-coli should be done in all cases of urinary infection or in the case of diarrhea. It includes testing the immune system (Al), lymphatic system (Ly), intestines (GI/LI, IG/SI), kidneys (R/KI), bladder (V/UB), and gallbladder (VB/GB).

Homeopathic remedies for E-coli, confirmed by Voll testing
No medicine for E-coli bacterium has been specified in the homeopathic literature yet. The best homeopathic remedies for E-coli found by Voll testing are: Acidum benzoicum, Acidum picricum, Arundo, Cantharis, Chininum arsenicum, Chromium kali sulphuricum, Kalium bromatum, Kalium iodatum, and Mercury salts (Table 3).

5.3.2.7. SALMONELLA

Salmonella bacteria belong to the family Enterobacteriaceae. The first type of Salmonella (S. choleraesuis) was found in 1885. There are 2,300 serotypes known nowadays. The most common are: S. enteritidis, S. gallinarum, S. paratyphi, S. typhi, S. typhimurium, and S. wichita. They are the main cause of enteric infections, such as typhoid fever, food poisoning with diarrhea, pain and tenderness in the abdomen. They are large bacteria, motile, with filaments. The infection is through the fecal–oral route and the bacteria can also be found in urine. The incubation period is from 6 hours to 10 days. The most severe infections can be found in infants, immune-suppressed individuals, and patients with sickle cell anemia. The bacteria can affect the intestines, liver, gallbladder, spleen, kidneys, bone marrow, and lymphoid tissue in the abdomen—in the Peyer's patches. Occasional complications can appear, such as acute suppurative periostitis and osteitis, reactive arthritis, abscess of the kidney, acute cholecystitis, and bronchopneumonia. Salmonella septicemia can occur and can affect every organ. Salmonella can persist in the body for more than a year after recovery from typhoid fever, and many individuals continue to be carriers for the remainder of their lives. The bacilli are most commonly present in the gallbladder and rarely in the urinary tract. The bacteria produce an endotoxin, a lipopolysaccharide. The following resonance vibrations for Salmonella bacteria are known from the research of Dr. H. Clark: 329 KHz, 365.05–371.1 KHz, 382.3–386.55 KHz [Clark, 1995]. Voll tests on Salmonella sufferers show that the most aggravating foods are: sugar, wheat, starch, and alcohol (Table 4).

EAV test for Salmonella

The EAV test for Salmonella must be carried out in all cases of diarrhea. The test should include immune and lymphatic systems (Al, Ly), intestines (GI/LI, IG/SI), gallbladder (VB/GB), liver (F/LV), spleen (RP/SP), kidneys (R/KI), and the meridian of the joints (Ad/JO).

Homeopathic remedies for Salmonella infection, confirmed by Voll testing

No specific homeopathic medicine for Salmonella bacteria is mentioned in the homeopathic literature. Testing with the Voll machine, we found that two remedies are useful in the case of Salmonella infection: Arsenicum album and Arsenicum iodatum. A good homeopathic remedy for Salmonella, according to Usupov [Usupov, 2000], is Veratrum album (Table 3).

5.3.2.8. ENTEROCOCCUS

Enterococcus is a bacterium originally classified in the group of Streptococci. A separate genus—Enterococci—was proposed in 1984. Enterococcus is a Gram-positive, oval bacterium, occurring singly, in pairs, or in short chains; and facultatively anaerobic, growing at 10–45°C (optimum 35°C). The bacterium is glucose-fermenting without gas production. It can occur anywhere: in soil, food, water, plants, animals, birds, and insects. The bacteria of the genus Enterococci are part of the gut flora in humans. When this flora's balance is disturbed, they can cause abdominal, skin, urinary tract, and bloodstream infections. There are many species of the genus Enterococcus: E. avium, E. casseliflavus, E. cecorum, E. gallinarum, E. hirae, E. mundtii, E. pseudovium, E. faecium, E. faecalis, E. saccharolyticus, E. sulphureus. About 80% of the infections are caused by E. faecalis. Enterococcus bacteria are known among the antibiotic-resistant bacteria. Their resistance to Penicillin, to Ampicillin, and to Vancomycin causes major concern about the treatment of this type of infection. Our research shows that the resonance vibration 325 KHz supports the immune system against Enterococcus. Increased oxygen in the blood is beneficial for treating the bacteria. Dairy products, sugar, and alcohol should be avoided in the case of Enterococcus infection (Table 4).

EAV detecting of Enterococcus
The meridians where Enterococcus can be detected are: the immune system (Al), large and small intestines (GI/LI, IG/SI), urogenital tract (R/KI,V/UB), and spleen (RP/SP).

Homeopathic remedies for Enterococcus confirmed by Voll testing
Remedies for this type of bacteria are not mentioned in the homeopathic literature. By Voll testing we found that the following homeopathic remedies are successful for Enterococcus infections: Arsenicum album, Arsenicum iodatum, Bryonia alba, Chininum arsenicum, Lycopodium, Natrium arsenicum, Phosphorus, and Sarsaparilla. The remedy Hydrastis canadensis is confirmed by Usupov [Usupov, 2000] (Table 3).

5.3.2.9. ENTEROBACTER (AEROBACTER) COLI

The bacteria Enterobacter are part of the bacterial flora of man. These bacteria depend on the family Enterobacteriaceae; Enterobacter bacteria and Coliform bacteria are often associated with E-coli. Enterobacter (Aerobacter) are Gram-negative rods, aerobes, and facultative anaerobes, and they inhabit the bowels, urinary tract, and respiratory tract. Those most often mentioned in the literature are: Enterobacter aerogenes and

Enterobacter cloacae. We find signals of these bacteria mainly in cases of chronic complaints of abdominal discomfort, bloated bowels, and heaviness after eating, with accumulation of fat around the waist. The EAV tests of food show that in Enterobacter cases the patient diet should exclude dairy, sugar, and fructose (Table 4). Our research found that the resonance vibration 374 KHz is helpful for the immune system in cases with these bacteria.

Homeopathic medicine for Enterobacter (Aerobacter), confirmed by Voll testing

Homeopathic remedies specific for these pathogens are not mentioned in the homeopathic literature. Our research by Voll testing showed the following remedies for Enterobacter (Aerobacter): Acidum picricum, Argentum nitricum, Arsenicum album, and Bryonia alba (Table 3).

5.3.2.10. PSEUDOMONAS

Pseudomonas are aerobic, Gram-negative, motile bacteria living in moist places in nature, as well as in kitchens, bathrooms, etc. They can inhabit insects and animals and can be found in soil and plants. The most commonly known are Pseudomonas aeruginosa, P. fluorescence, P. geniculata, and P. pyocyaneus. In man these bacteria can cause infections of the urinary tract, lungs, infected ulcers or bedsores, cornea ulcerations, otitis externa, and other infections. These bacteria can cause infections in hospitals. The resonance frequencies discovered by Dr. H. Clark for Pseudomonas aeruginosa are: 331.25–334.6 KHz [Clark, 1995]. We found that 406 KHz works as well. A food test usually shows intolerance to dairy products and sugar (Table 4).

Homeopathic remedies for Pseudomonas, confirmed by Voll testing

We found two homeopathic remedies for Pseudomonas by Voll test: China and Bryonia (Table 3).

5.3.2.11. BORRELIA

Borrelia bacteria belong to the genus of Spirochaetes. Under dark field microscopy they look like large, motile, prolonged bodies with multiple fibrils. Borrelia duttonii bacterium can be transmitted by lice and ticks. It causes fever, known as African relapsing fever and European relapsing fever. The infection can affect the spleen, liver, kidneys, and brain. Borrelia vincentii causes ulcerative gingivostomatitis. The resonance frequences for Borrelia according to Dr. Clark are 378.95–382.0 KHz [Clark, 1995].

Homeopathic medicine for Borrelia confirmed by Voll testing
We found one good working homeopathic remedy for Borrelia by Voll testing: Arsenicum iodatum (Table 3).

5.3.2.12. BRUCELLA

Brucella are Gram-negative bacilli, round like cocci, non-motile, non-sporing, and non-capsulate. They remain alive in the soil, they live in animals and affect man as well, causing acute attacks or chronic brucellosis, known as Mediterranean fever or Malta fever. The most often recognized are: B. abortus—in cattle, B. melitensis—in goats and sheep, B. suis—in pigs, B. ovis—affecting genitals. All of them affect man. The infection can be detected in the immune system, liver, spleen, and bones. We found one case by official diagnosis of chronic Brucellosis affecting the heart.

Homeopathic remedies for Brucella, confirmed by Voll testing
We found two homeopathic remedies for Brucella by Voll testing: Colchicum and Causticum. Usupov [Usupov, 2000] confirmed the remedy Cardius marianus (Table 3).

5.3.2.13. PROTEUS

Proteus bacteria are Gram-negative, actively motile rods, classified in the family of the Enterobacteriaceae together with E-coli, Salmonella, Shigella, Enterobacter, and Serratia. They are facultative anaerobes. They ferment sugars in anaerobic conditions, but can use a wide range of organic substances in aerobic conditions. Proteus species are mainly soil inhabitants, decomposing organic mater [Deacon]. Proteus vulgaris is most commonly known as a pathogen bacterium, causing urinary tract infections with high alkalizing of the urine. It degrades urea to ammonia by the production of the enzyme urease, and it can cause sediments of the type Calcium Phosphoricum in the urinary tract. Proteus mirabilis is known to cause summer diarrhea in infants. According to the research of Dr. H. Clark, the characteristic resonance frequencies for the genus Proteus are: 320.55–326.0 KHz; 327.2–329.5 KHz; 333.75–339.15 KHz, 345.95–352.1 KHz; and 408.75–416.45 KHz [Clark, 1995]. In the case of a Proteus infection, the EAV food test shows intolerance to sugar, fructose, dairy products, and alcohol (Table 4).

Homeopathic remedies for Proteus confirmed by Voll testing

By Voll test we found the following homeopathic remedies for balancing the signal from Proteus bacteria: Acidum nitricum, Aurum iodatum, Aurum metallicum, Aurum muriaticum, Clematis, Mezereum, Phosphorus, Pyrogenium, and Sepia. According to Usupov [Usupov, 2000], a good remedy for Proteus is Cinnabaris (Table 3).

5.3.2.14. SHIGELLA

Shigella are Gram-negative, motile bacteria of the family Enterobacteriaceae. The species S. sonnei, S. flexneri, S. boydii, S. dysenteriae, and S. paradysenteriae have a pathogenic capacity for man, causing diarrhea, colic, fever, and abdominal pain. The bacteria affect the epithelial cells of the colon and causes capillary thrombosis leading to blood in the stool, i.e. bloody diarrhea. Neurotoxins are produced during the growth and spread of the bacteria. The source of the infection could be food, water, or even direct contact between children in daycare groups. [Dupont, 1995]. The best way to prevent this type of infection is to improve the hygiene in the kitchen and to wash hands regularly. According to Dr. H. Clark, the specific resonance frequencies for Shigella bacteria are: 318.0 KHz; 390.089 KHz; and 394.0 KHZ [Clark, 1995]. In the case of Shigella infection, taking antioxidants is beneficial for the immune system. The diet should exclude sugar, fructose, and dairy products (Table 4).

Homeopathic medicine for Shigella, confirmed by Voll testing

Medicine for Shigella bacteria is not specified in the homeopathic literature. We found some good remedies by Voll testing: Carbo vegetabilis,

Chininum arsenicum, Cuprum aceticum, and Cuprum metallicum (Table 3).

5.3.2.15. TUBERCULOSIS PATHOGENS

For detecting the pathogens of tuberculosis, the following homeopathic nosodes are used: Tuberculinum-Coch (Tub-Coch), Tuberculinum-bovinum (Tub-bov), and Tuberculinum-avis (Tub- avis). All of them are important for testing, because they correspond to different types of Mycobacterium tuberculosis in man: M. tuberculosis, M. bovis, M. avium. They are curved rods 3 μm × 0.3 μm, in size, single or in pairs, and slow-growing. Usually they do not survive more than 20 min at 60°C or if exposed to sunlight. But they have been found in small numbers in pasteurized milk. Most often species of Mycobacterium invade the lungs, but many other organs could be affected. Mycobacterium avium subspecies para-tuberculosis (MAP) is taught to be responsible for many cases of Crohn's disease in the digestive system, according to Professor John Hermon-Taylor from the UK [Zinger, 2003]. Other types of Mycobacterium can cause illness in man:

M. kansasii can affect the lungs of man in industrial areas, often found in the UK; M. intracellulare affects the lungs (Battey bacillus); M. xenopi affects the lungs, often in South Africa; M. smegmatis affects the genitals; M. fortuitum is found in fish, amphibians, and reptiles, but in man can cause abscesses in the lungs and the lymph glands; and M. ulcerans and M. marinum live in fish and amphibians, but in man can cause skin infections, known as Buruly ulcer in Uganda, and affects arms and legs.

According to Professor G. Enderlein [Enderlein, 1916], the bacteria of the group Mycobacterium tuberculosis are connected with the fungus Aspergillus. He considers that Aspergillus niger is the higher degree in the development of Mycobacteria, as one of its polymorphic forms which appear with changes of conditions in the internal environment (milieu). That is why lifestyle and food intake are important for the development of tuberculosis. Mycobacterium species are closely connected with AIDS, according to L. Broxmeyer [Broxmeyer, 2003]. An active process of tuberculosis is indicated by symptoms such as a febrile condition, perspiration, loss of weight, weakness, coughing, and blood in the mucous. Tuberculosis bacilli can spread all over the body and can affect different

146

organs. For patients with a compromised immune system, tuberculosis can be deadly dangerous. Many people can be infected without obvious symptoms, but they can spread the infection by coughing and sneezing. The conventional treatment with antibiotics is becoming more and more difficult, because of the resistance of the bacteria to many of them.

EAV testing for pathogens causing tuberculosis

The EAV test for Mycobacterium tuberculosis begins with measurements of the meridian of the immune system. The point Al-6 usually shows inflammation of the lungs. The meridian of the lungs (P/ LU) has to be tested on the left and right sides. It is essential to test with different testers for the different types of tuberculosis pathogens mentioned above. The meridians of the bowels (GI/ LI; IG/SI) and of the spleen (RP/ SP) are often involved, showing the infection.

Specific frequencies for these pathogens are, according to H. Clark [Clark, 1995], 409.65–410.65 KHz and 430.55–434.2 KHz. These are useful for supporting the vibrational energy of the immune system.

Homeopathic remedies for tuberculosis

Many homeopathic remedies are used for tuberculosis: Agar, Calc, Calc-p., Hep., Iod., Kali-c., Kali-s., Lyc., Phos., Psor., Puls., Sil., Spong., Stann., Sulph., Ther., Tub., Zinc, and others [Murphy, 1996].

Homeopathic remedies for tuberculosis confirmed by Voll testing

Usupov confirmed by Voll testing the remedies Kreosotum and Scrofularia [Usupov, 2000]. Our experience shows that the best is the mix of Tuberculinum nosodes, combined with Mercury salts or with Phosphorus. Very often the remedies listed for the fungi Aspergillus work well (Table 3).

5.3.2.16. MYCOPLASMA AND UREAPLASMA

Mycoplasma is a genus of small prokaryotic cells, about 300×125 nm in size. Their colonies can be seen with a light microscope. Mycoplasma can cause 20% to 40% of the cases of pneumonia. In the genus Mycoplasma, there are a number of species: M. arthritidis, M. fermentance, M. hominis, M. pneumoniae, and very closely related to them is Ureaplasma urealyticus. M. pneumonia is the most common, causing febrile bronchitis or pneumonia with myalgia, sore throat, headache, and cough. The cough is usually a dry, nonproductive deep one. Sometimes the condition is combined with nausea and vomiting. The complications can include skin rashes, ear infections, meningitis, encephalitis, arthritis, and hemolytic anaemia. Mycoplasma can cause ovarian abscesses, salpingitis, puerperal sepsis, hemorrhagic cystitis, and urethritis. Ureaplasma urealyticum affects the urogenital tract of man. A large part of nonspecific urethritis tested negative to Chlamydia can be due to Ureaplasma. It can be the cause of repeated spontaneous abortions, can give pain in the bladder and vagina, and in some cases can be involved in Reiter's syndrome. M. fermentans and M. arthritidis affect the joints causing rheumatoid arthritis. These microorganisms are carbohydrate-fermenting. That is why in the case of Mycoplasma and Ureaplasma infections it is advisable to stop the intake of sugar (glucose and fructose). As a result of their function, Ureaplasma splits urea to ammonium, and M. arthritidis splits amino acids such as arginine to ammonium. Mycoplasma and Ureaplasma belong to a group of cell-wall–deficient bacteria. This was confirmed by the research group of V. Livingston in the US. As the action of most of the antibiotics is by destroying the cell walls of the bacteria, it is difficult to treat Mycoplasma infections with antibiotics. That is why any new and different approach to controlling Mycoplasma and Ureaplasma deserves attention.

EAV testing for Mycoplasma and Ureaplasma pathogens

The EAV test can detect Mycoplasma and Ureaplasma in the immune system meridian (Al), lymphatic system (Ly), lungs (P/LU), spleen (RP/SP), bladder (V/UB), kidneys (R/KI), and other organs. The food test usually shows that the diet should exclude sugar, fructose, soy, vinegar, and alcohol (Table 4). Specific resonance vibrations for Mycoplasma pathogens are 322.85–323.9 and 342.75–349.30 [Clark, 1995]. They can be used to boost the immune system at that part of the energy spectrum. Vitamin B complex, Vitamin C, and antioxidants are useful, helping the spleen to return to its normal condition (the test is on RP/SP, left side).

Homeopathic remedies for Mycoplasma and Ureaplasma infections confirmed by Voll testing

Specific remedies for these types of infections are not recommended in homeopathic repertories.

By EAV test we found the following homeopathic remedies: Arsenicum album, Arsenicum iodatum, Chlorinum, Graphites, Kalium arsenicum, Kalium bromatum, Kalium carbonicum, Kalium iodatum, Kalium phosphoricum, Phosphorus, Pyrogenium, Spongia, and Sticta (Table 3).

5.3.2.17. KLEBSIELLA

Klebsiella is a genus of saprophytic bacteria. It can be found in natural water, in human and animal intestines, in the urinary tract, in the lungs and upper respiratory tract. It can be a source of infection in hospitals. The bacteria live in colonies visible under a light microscope. There are 72 species of Klebsiella. The most common species are: Kl. aerogenes, Kl. pneumoniae, Kl. edvardsii, Kl. rhinoseromatis, and Kl. ozena.

Klebsiella causes a chronic granulomatosis condition with lesions of the mucous membranes. Very often the infection is in the lungs, nose, throat, and mouth. The joints can be affected with arthritis and deformations. Klebsiella produce gas from glucose and acids from lactose. In the case of Klebsiella infection, the EAV food test shows intolerance to sugar, fructose, and dairy products (Table 4).

The resonance vibrations useful for the immune system in Klebsiella infection are in the following spectral area: 398.45–404.65 KHz and 416.9–421.9 KHz [Clark, 1995]. Vitamin C and antioxidants are beneficial in cases of Klebsiella infection.

EAV test for Klebsiella species

The EAV test includes Immune system (Al), Lymphatic system (Ly), Lungs (P/LU), and the signal can be detected in the meridian of the joints (Ad/JO). In more serious infections, the spleen (RP/SP) is also involved.

149

Homeopathic remedies for Klebsiella bacteria, confirmed by Voll testing

There are no specific homeopathic remedies for Klebsiella in the repertories. By EAV test we found the remedies Antimonium tartaricum, Arsenicum album, Lobelia, and Sticta pulmonaria to be beneficial for Klebsiella (Table 3).

5.3.2.18. STAPHYLOCOCCUS

Staphylococcus is a genus of spherical bacteria the size of 1 μm in diameter, grouped in round, grape-like colonies. The bacteria produce acids from glucose. There are many different species: Staphylococcus aureus, Staph. albus, Micrococcus, Peptococcus. Staph. aureus can be found in the skin causing acne, abscesses, and wound infections; it can affect nose, throat, lungs, and bronchi with bronchopneumonia; it can cause acute food poisoning with enterocolitis; or it can cause osteomyelitis, pyelonephritis, lymphadenitis, endocarditis, and other infections. Staphylococcus is now one of the most resistant bacteria to antibiotics. In 1945, it was found that about 14% of Staph. aureus bacteria were resistant to Penicillin, according to Dr. G. Fleming, the discoverer of this antibiotic. By 1995, already 95% of these bacteria were resistant, and this created a huge question about the use of antibiotics for Staphylococcus infections. In the case of Staphylococcus infection, the allergy test by the Voll machine shows intolerance to dairy, sugar, and alcohol (Table 4). The spectral area of the vibrations useful for supporting the immune system in the case of Staphylococcus infection is: 376.27–381.00 KHz [Clark, 1995].

EAV detecting of Staphylococcus bacteria

The EAV test should start with the meridians of the immune system (Al), lymphatic system (Ly), and spleen (RP/SP). Many other organs can show signals for these bacteria, but the best for testing the right medicine are the above-mentioned meridians.

Homeopathic remedies for Staphylococcus

According to the R. Murphy Repertory, the main homeopathic remedies for Staphylococcus are: Antimonium crudum, Arsenicum album,

150

Arsenicum iodatum, Calcarea carbonica, Carbo animalis, Carbo vegetabilis, Causticum, Cicuta, Clematis, Conium, Crotalus horridus, Dulcamara, Echinacea, Hepar sulphur, Iris versicolor, Kalium bichromicum, Kreosotum, Lycopodium, Mercurius solubilis, Natrium muriaticum, Acidum nitricum, Acidum phosphoricum, Phosphorus, Pyrogenium, Rhus toxicodendron, Sarsaparilla, Sepia, Silicea, Staphysagria, Sulphur, and Viola tricolor [Murphy, 1996].

Homeopathic remedies for Staphylococcus confirmed by Voll testing
By Voll testing for Staphylococcus, we found the following homeopathic remedies: Antimonium arsenicum, Chininum arsenicum, Coffea, Hepar sulphuricum, Kalium bichromicum, and Mercury salts. The work of Usupov [Usupov, 2000] shows the remedies Cactus, Convolaria, Phytolacca, Strophanthus, and Silica as confirmed by Voll testing (Table 3). More oxygen in the body helps the immune system in the case of Staphylococcus infection.

5.3.2.19. STREPTOCOCCUS

Streptococcus bacteria are spherical in shape, about 1 μm in diameter, living in chain-like colonies, and easily distinguished under a light microscope. Most of the species are facultatively anaerobic, they can live in aerobic and anaerobic conditions; some of the species are strictly anaerobic. There are many different types of Streptococcus. The most common are: Str. pyogenes, Str. viridans, Str. faecalis, Aerococcus, Pneumococcus, Str. mutans. They cause tonsillitis, pharyngitis, sinusitis, otitis media, bronchopneumonia, meningitis, glomerulonephritis, scarlet fever, rheumatic fever, skin infections, dental caries, abscesses, and many other serious conditions. The treatment of Streptococcus is now more and more difficult due to its resistance to most of the antibiotics. Streptococcus is a parasitic type of microorganism, it thrives on readily available amino acids. This results in the idea that during a Streptococcus infection the intake of proteins should be reduced. In the case of Streptococcus infection, the food test often shows intolerance to dairy products, sugar, and alcohol (Table 4). The spectral area of vibration energy helping the immune system in the case of Streptococcus infections is between 313 and 387 KHz: 313.8–321.1; 360.5–375.3; 366.85–370.2; 368.15–368.85; and 382–387 KHz [Clark, 1995].

EAV detecting of Streptococcus bacteria

The EAV test can find Streptococcus signals in various organs. It is essential to test the immune system (Al), lymphatic system (Ly), liver (F/LV), and kidneys (R/KI). A signal from the spleen (RP/SP) is usually a sign that the infection is more serious.

Homeopathic remedies for Streptococcus bacteria

According to the R. Murphy Repertory, the homeopathic remedies for Streptococcus are:

Acidum sulphuricum, Ailanthus, Arnica, Arsenicum album, Belladonna, Streptococcus, and X-ray [Murphy, 1996].

Homeopathic remedies for Streptococcus, confirmed by Voll testing

By EAV testing we confirmed the action of the following homeopathic remedies: Acidum sulphuricum, Arsenicum album, Kali arsenicum, Mercurius cyanatus, Mercurius solubilis, Mercurius vivus, Phosphorus, Pulsatilla, Rhus toxicodendron, and Sticta pulmonaria. Usupov [Usupov, 2000] confirmed the following remedies: Crataegus, Dioscorea, Phytolacca, and Urtica urens (Table 3).

5.3.3. EAV AND HOMEOPATHY FOR FUNGAL INFECTIONS

The fungi are classified as Oomycetes. They are microscopic creatures in between plants and animals, closer to the group of Protozoa. They are divided into four groups:

- Molds with vegetative mycelium;
- Yeast that are unicellular spherical cells, budding new cells;
- Yeast-like that grow partly as yeast, partly as long filamentous cells, named pseudomycelium;
- Dimorphic fungi which develop in the form of yeast or mycelium depending on the environmental conditions such as temperature, acidity (pH), and others.

5.3.3.1. PLEOMORPHIC THEORY
OF PROFESSOR G. ENDERLEIN

The subject of pathogenic fungi cannot be considered separately from the new ideas in microbiology developed by Professor G. Enderlein [Enderlein, 1916], during the period from 1914 to 1968.

The theory is radical and disputable, because it contradicts the fundamental postulates of the microbiology of Louis Pasteur, studied nowadays in all universities. This theory may be the beginning of a revolution in biology and medicine in the next few decades. The main conclusions of the research of Enderlein are summarized by Dr. Maria Bleker [Bleker, 1993], a follower of his discoveries, practicing dark field microscopy of live blood:

1. *"The cell is not the smallest living unit, but the colloid is."* The colloids are below visibility by the light microscope, less than 20 nm.

2. *"The proof that bacteria have nuclei or nucleic equivalents (Mych)..."* It became confirmed (Harmsen) through the development of phase contrast and the electron microscope.

3. *"Proof of the sexual propagation of bacteria... Nonsexual propagation occurs by sprouting and splitting, the sexual is connected copulation or nucelic fusion.* Sexual propagation has been confirmed by the research of Nobel Prize recipient J. Lederberg, US, El-Taumg, US, and W. Hayes, Edinburgh, UK."

4. *"The scientific proof of Pleomorphism in microbes.* This teaching reveals that a certain type of microbe can occur in diverse forms and developmental stages under precisely established conditions, beginning with the smallest particles of ultramicroscopic magnitudes up to the large, multinucleic, highly developed stages of bacteria and fungi... All this has been confirmed through research done in more recent years by the Tuberculosis Research Institute in Borstel, Germany, by G. Kolbel, D. Domagk, S. Uyeda, H. Harmsen, and G. Meinecke."

5. *"The proof that there is no sterile, germ-free blood.* Enderlein says that in the serum of all people and warm-blooded animals there are living microorganisms. He called them Endobionts. . . . Enderlein revealed that there is a developmental form of the Endobionts which is of plant nature. He called them Thecits and recognized them to be entirely identical with thrombocytes. . . . It has also become confirmed that English researchers have certified plant enzymes to be on trombocytes."

6. *"The human being lives in symbiosis with a plant microorganism, the Endobiont." Everybody receives this microorganism via ovum, sperm, and placenta from their parents.* The lower stages of the development of the Endobiont are apathogenic and therapeutically useful. The advanced stages of the Endobiont can facilitate or produce degenerative disease. According to Enderlein, the main cause of the development of the higher stage of the Endobiont is over-acidification of the blood. The healthiest pH of blood is 7.35. Any acidification leads to the development of higher and more harmful stages of the Endobiont. There are many conditions, caused by civilization, that aggravate the biochemistry of man: the exposure to strong electromagnetic fields, radiation, special gases that kill the normal ecosystem on Earth, food intake of too much protein and sugar, our internal environment polluted with heavy metals, insecticides, and nitrites, and the uncontrolled use of medical drugs. These lead to a serious disturbance of the biochemical equilibrium in our bodies.

7. *"Disease means symbiotic disturbance."* The steps to health are steps to symbiotic balance.

8. *Pleomorphically considered, all microbes have their natural cycle of development, beginning with the Primitive phase, changing to the Bacterial phase, and finally culminating in the Fungal phase. The fungal culmination can also be replaced by Yeast culmination.*

9. *This teaching reveals that the microbes can occur in diverser forms and developmental stages. The Fungal phase has two forms: Aspergillus niger and Mucor racemosus.* Aspergillus niger is connected with the

bacterial form causing tuberculosis, and its fungal form can be seen in the blood by dark field examination in cases of diabetes, rheumatoid arthritis, and other degenerative diseases. Mucor racemosus is connected with the bacterial form Propionibacterium acnes, and its fungal form can be seen in the blood by dark field microscopy in hypoxic conditions, cerebral–cardiovascular disseminations, and degenerative diseases.

Only time will show if Enderelein's theory will prevail. The fact is that so many people are very acidic and their organisms need alkalizing. The other fact is that so many patients tested by EAV show the presence of pathogenic fungi, especially those with chronic and degenerative diseases and weak immune systems. To detect the pathogens and to apply the proper homeopathic medicine means to supply the immune system with the quantum energy frequencies it needs at that moment. On the basis of the discoveries of Enderlein in Germany, the medical company Sanum has produced various new medicines.

5.3.3.2. THE MOST COMMON PATHOGENIC FUNGI

There are many different fungal pathogens. We will consider only a few of them, that is those most important for human pathogenesis.

5.3.3.2.1. ASPERGILLUS

The genus Aspergillus includes filamentous fungi, i.e. molds that are yellow, green, or black in color. The most common are: A. fisheri, A. flavus, A. fumigatus, A. niger, A. orizae, A. terrens, and A. versicolor. A. fumigatus and A. niger are known to cause abortions in cattle and lung disease in man, aspergillosis. It can be an allergic form in asthmatic patients with a reaction to the inhalation of spores (sensitization) with allergic alveolitis; the colonization form in individuals with a previous lung condition, when a fungus ball (aspergilloma) can be formed in an existing cavity; or the third form: dissemination of the fungus throughout the body. The fungus can invade sinuses, ears, gastrointestinal tract, and can cause ophthalmic infections. When it invades the blood vessels, it can cause thrombosis and may lodge in the brain, heart, and kidneys [Mackie & McCartney, 1978].

155

5.3.3.2.2. MUCOR

Mucor fungi belong to the genus Mucoracea. They are common saprophytic molds. The most common species are M. corymbifera, M. mucedo, M. plumbeus, and M. racemosus. In nature they live on dead and decaying organic materials. They invade man causing chronic infections of the lungs, bronchi, and mucous membranes of the nose and sinuses. Many cases of invasive fungal sinusitis (IFS) caused by Mucor mycosis are reported by medical researchers in Atlanta, Georgia, US. Mucor could be dangerous for patients with blood malignancy, systemic chemotherapy, diabetes, and patients on chronic systemic steroid treatment [Parikh, Venkataraman, & DelGaudio, 2004]. Mucor can invade the mucosa of the intestines. Any segment of the gastrointestinal tract can be affected with erosive ulcers and thrombosis or gangrene [Groves, 1998]. Mycosis of the ears caused by Mucor is very common [Mackie & McCartney, 1978]. Mucor can be the cause of various problems of the cardiovascular system with sclerosis, thrombosis, and infarcts. Mucor can be expressed as skin diseases, of which the most serious is a disseminated disease in patients with neutropenia and diabetes with ketoacidosis, in the cases of immunosuppressed or immunocompromised patients [Groves, 1998].

5.3.3.2.3. CANDIDA

The genus Candida belongs to the group of Yeast-like fungi, growing partly like yeast with budding cells 250–400 nm in diameter and producing 700–1700 nm long tubular cells referred to as pseudomycelium. Candida ferments carbohydrates, it cannot split urea. This is important when considering the diet: Any sugar and starch intake can feed Candida, but proteins are allowed. There are about 100 species of Candida. The most commonly known are: C. albicans, C. tropicalis, C. pseudotropicalis, C. parapsilosis, C. krusei, C. lusitaniae, C. glabrata, C. stellatoidea, and others. Candida affects the mucus membranes of the mouth, throat, and sinuses. Very often it grows in the vagina causing thrush. It can cause skin problems with itchy skin in the folds. The effect of Candida on the digestive system is serious. The invasion has many different aspects such as malnutrition, leaky gut syndrome, allergic reactions, and toxification.

Candida can affect the lungs and kidneys as a secondary infection, according to Mackie and McCartney [Mackie & McCartney, 1978] and Trowbridge and Walker [Trowbridge & Walker, 1986]. Systemic Candidiasis, which is an invasion of the whole human body, can occur, and it is a sign of a weak immune system. Candida organisms excrete toxic substances.The filamentous tubes of the germ are especially toxic, invading deeply into the tissue of the mucosa of the gut, kidney tissue, lungs, and the lining of the vagina. The toxins are oxidants. That is why the intake of antioxidants is part of the treatment. There are many different causative effects of our civilized life that trigger the invasion of fungi and Candida:

- Increased and uncontrolled use of antibiotics which reduces the total population level of the indigenous bacterial flora, killing the friendly bacteria of the gut such as Lactobacillus acidophilus and L. bifidus.
- Antibiotics in animal feed stimulate Candidiasis in humans.
- Oral contraceptive pills stimulate Candida, and that is why many young women suffer from a Candida infection.
- Corticosteroid chronic medications used often even for children increases the growth of Candida.
- Low biochemical quality of food consumed in civilized countries causes nutritional deficiencies and increases the aggressiveness of Candida, which then develops its toxic tubular form.
- Toxic substances and pollutants in the air and in the water promote the yeast syndrome. Insecticides, herbicides, aerosol sprays, detergents, and disinfectants for home care, motor vehicle products, solvents, and plastics all irritate the immune system.
- Of particular importance are the heavy metals from tooth fillings which are one of the main reasons for persistent yeast infections in the body.

The symptoms of Candida infection fit a broad spectrum: digestive discomfort, bloated abdomen from various foods, especially from bread, milk, sugar, alcohol, beer, and cheese. At the same time, the person experiences craving for sweets, chocolate, and sweet drinks, and puts on weight around the waistline. Puffiness, water retention, and irritation in the respiratory system and in the urinary tract; vaginal discharge and itchiness are also experienced. Very often the main complaints are fatigue, lethargy, a drowsy mental state, and headaches. Menstrual irregularities, premenstrual tension, irritability, and sudden weakness are other common symptoms. The general feeling is as if something is producing poisons in the body all the time, which is what Candida does.

Homeopathic remedies for Candida infections, confirmed by Voll test:

Acidum carbolicum, Acidum fluoricum, Acidum lacticum, Acidum picricum, Aurum iodatum, Bellis perennis, Borax, Phosphorus, and Pyrogen (Table 3).

These homeopathic remedies are given in combination with the supporting natural supplements, after the latter have been tested.

5.3.3.2.4. CRYPTOCOCCUS

The genus Cryptococcus is a member of the Yeast family. It includes 37 species. The fungal spores of Cryptococcus are common in soil and can be breathed in with dust. It can affect man, and domestic animals such as dogs, cats, goats, and birds. Cryptococcus is found in the droppings of pigeons. Cryptococcus neoformans is pathogenic to man. It makes rapidly growing colonies of round, budding yeast cells. The colonies can be creamy, slightly pink, or yellowish to brown in color. C. neoformans is known to affect the lungs, skin, prostate gland, urinary tract, eyes, myocardium, bones, and joints. The most serious effect is on the central nervous system, especially the brain, causing meningitis and meningoencephalitis. The intensity of the Cryptococcal infection definitely depends on the status of the immune system. Many people have unknowingly been exposed to the fungus with no serious effects. For patients with a compromised immune system (often AIDS patients), Cryptococcal meningoencephalitis is a serious opportunistic infection causing damage to the neural cells and the gray matter of the brain. The symptoms of Cryptococcal meningitis and meningoencephalitis can be fever, nausea, vomiting, visual problems, severe headache with pressure, neurological symptoms, sometimes seizures, stiff neck, fatigue, and a general feeling of being unwell. For controlling this infection, Amphotericin B intravenous injections and the pills Fluconazole (Diflucan) are used, which have serious side effects and cannot be used for a long period of time.

5.3.3.2.5. DERMATOPHYTES

The Dermatophytes are fungi metabolizing the keratin of the skin, hair, and nails. This infection can affect individuals who are otherwise healthy. Most affected are exhausted patients with weakened immune systems. There are three groups of Dermatophytes: Trichophyton affecting skin, nails, and hair, Microsporum affecting skin and hair, and Epidermophyton affecting skin and nails. These are the fungi which cause ringworm (Tinea): Tinea pedis—feet, Tinea capitis—scalp, Tinea manuum —hands, Tinea cruris—groin and genital area. The most common species are: Trichophyton tonsurans, T. rubrum, T. violaceum, T. schoenleinii. T. megninii, T. soudanense, Microsporum audouinii, M. ferrugineum, and Epidermophyton floccosum. Many Dermatophytes are zoophilic, that is they affect domestic animals. In cases of mycosis of the skin, some yeast species such as Malassezia furfur and Candida can also be responsible [Mycology of Dermatophyte Infections].

EAV testing for fungal pathogens

The test for fungal pathogens starts with the immune system, and the point Al-1 is most important for detecting Candida infection. Very often only this point is enough to detect Candida in the gut. The meridian of the lymphatic system (Ly) will indicate whether the fungus is in the mucus membranes of the nose and sinuses. It is advisable to test the lungs (P/ LU), bladder (V/UB), kidneys (R/KI), and intestines (GI/LI, IG/SI) also. For all fungal infections, it is important to test the spleen (RP/SP). The substances to be used for supporting the immune system are usually tested in the meridian of the spleen. Any other complaints have to be taken into consideration, and the other often-affected meridians can be joints (Ad/Jo), nerves (Nd/NE), liver (F/LV), hormones (TR/TW), and circulation (MC/ CI). It is essential to test a salt with alkaline properties such as bicarbonate of soda ($NaHCO_3$), because in most of the cases of fungal infections the body system is very acidic. In the case of Candida, it is necessary to test for antioxidants. Non-acidic Vitamin C and Beta carotene are compulsory in the recommended Candida treatment. For infants we suggest fresh carrot juice with bio-flora and Vitamin C powder to be given twice a day. For many types of fungi, a good balance in the meridian system is achieved by using oxygen, ozone, and oxidants. Preparations containing good bio-flora such as Lactobacillus acidophilus and L. bifidus bacteria are part of the measures for restoring the balance in the gut. It is better to test preparations from different producers, so as to find the best one for the client. The resonance frequencies useful for treating the fungal pathogens are: 184 KHz, 325 KHz, 353 KHz, 365 KHz, 378 KHz, 385 KHz, 392 KHz, and 420 KHz. There could be many more frequencies that will be discovered with future research.

Homeopathic remedies for fungal infections

According to the R. Murphy Repertory [Murphy, 1996], there are many good remedies for treating fungi:

p. 425. Mycosis—Calcarea carbonica, Calcarea silicata, Graphytes, and Silicea.

p. 409. Fungus—Apis, Bacillinum, Calcarea iodata, Calcarea phosphorica, Phosphorus, Silicea, and Thuja.

p. 382. Actinomycosis—Hecla lava, Hippozaenium, Kalium iodatum, and Nitricum acidum.

p. 443. Tinea, general—Ailantus, Argentum nitricum, Calcarea carbonica, Carbo animalis, Carboneum sulphuratum, Carbo vegetabilis, China, Cina, Cuprum metallicum, Cuprum aceticum, Curare, Filix mas, Formica rufa, Fragaria, Granatum, Graphites, Gratiola, Kalium carbonicum, Kalium iodatum, Magnesium muriaticum, Mercurius solubilis, Natrium carbonicum, Natrium sulphuricum, Nux vomica, Petroleum, Phosphorus, Platinum, Pulsatilla, Sabadilla, Santoninum, Sepia, Silicea, Stannum, Sulphur, Terridion, Thuja, and Valeriana.

p. 616. Fungus, toes—Acidum nitricum, Antimonium crudum, Graphites, Sanicula, Sepia, Silicea, Thuja, and Zincum metallicum.

p. 422. Lichen planus—Agaricus muscarius, Anacardium, Antimonium crudum, Apis, Arsenicum album, Arsenicum iodatum, Chininum arsenicosum, Iodium, Juglans cinerea, Kalium bichromicum, Kalium iodatum, Ledum, Mercurius solubilis, Sarsaparilla, Staphysagria, and Sulphur iodatum.

p. 1444. Mouth, Thrush—Arum triphyllum, Borax, Iodium, Lac caninum, Kalium chloratum, Mercurius solubilis, Mercurius cyanatus, Muriaticum acidum, Natrium muriaticum, Nitricum acidum, Sanguinaria,

Sulphur, Sulphuricum acidum, Syphilinum, Thuja.

Homeopathic remedies for fungal infections confirmed by Voll testing
The homeopathic remedies that produce the best results for fungal pathogens that we found by Voll testing are: Acidum benzoicum, Acidum carbolicum, Acidum fluoricum, Acidum lacticum, Acidum nitricum, Acidum picricum, Acidum phosphoricum, Acidum sarcolacticum, Acidum sulphuricum, Aurum metallicum, Aurum muriaticum, Aurum iodatum, Arsenicum album, Arsenicum iodatum, Bellis perennis, Bismuthum metallicum, Bismuthum subnitricum, Borax, Bryonia, Causticum, Kalium iodatum, Mercurius solubilis, Phosphorus, and Pyrogenium (Table 3).

5.3.4. EAV AND HOMEOPATHY FOR VIRAL INFECTIONS

Viral infections and their treatment have always been a serious medical problem. Viruses are intracellular pathogens, so it is not possible to destroy them by destroying the host cells. This would be analogous to burning down the house because we have seen an insect in the cupboard.

The best approach is to boost the energy of the immune system, so that the energy level of the system is high and the virus cannot multiply. The measures include cleaning procedures, regulation of the red-oxy potential, regulation of the acidity (pH) and the concentration of salts in the liquids of the body so as to make sure that there is adequate nutrition for the cells. In other words, we have to improve the internal environment, the milieu of the system.

In conventional medicine, vitamins, boosters of the immune system, and antibiotics for preventing secondary infections are prescribed. At present it is difficult to offer antiviral drugs free of side effects. The laboratory diagnosis by blood tests is both costly and time-consuming. It is also not absolutely reliable. The blood tests are positive only when the infection is advanced. In a large number of cases the blood tests are negative, but the pathogen is there in a dormant condition, "an occult disease," according to winner of the Nobel Prize for medicine Charles Nicolle.

The emergence of another pathogen, or stress, or exhaustion, or an emotional problem can activate this agent and turn the condition into the symptomatic stage. This is especially important for intracellular pathogens such as viruses, which are capable of staying hidden in our cells.

In dark field microscopy of live blood, a viral condition can be seen as an increased number of lymphocytes with a dull gray appearance. Enlarged membranes, distorted nuclei, and bright inclusions are also signs of viral presence. Increased lymphocytes are seen in the blood of people with chronic fatigue syndrome, herpes, HIV, and Cytomegalo virus. It is not possible to differentiate which virus is present by dark field microscopy [Fredericks, 2001].

In iridology, if a dark spot is seen in the area of the spleen, the practitioner–iridologist may conclude that a chronic infection affecting the spleen is present. Differentiation of the pathogen is not possible.

The investigation of viruses requires a powerful electron microscope because the size of viruses is 20 to 300 nm (by comparison, Staphylococcus bacterium is 1,000 nm and E-coli bacterium is 3,000 nm). Very often serious and chronic viral infections are not diagnosed for years and many people spend their lives tired, lethargic, suffering with headaches, anemia, infertility, or developing serious chronic conditions such as pancreatitis, liver and kidney infections, or inflammations of lymphatic, thyroid, adrenal, and reproductive glands. That is why another viral testing method such as Electro Acupuncture by Voll is beneficial. A physical, noninvasive method such as the Voll test and the gentle treatment with homeopathic remedies, together with natural products for boosting the immune system, produce a good chance of a humane and intelligent recovery from viral infections.

The symptoms of chronic viral infection

Patients with chronic viral infections often have one major complaint: chronic fatigue. They are tired, sleepy, and exhausted even after long hours of sleep. They go to bed early, but in the morning are not fresh. Lack of enthusiasm, depression, panic attacks, and dissatisfaction are often manifested. On a physical level there are often flu-like symptoms, pain in the muscles and joints, headaches, periodically swollen glands, perspiration at night, persistent febrile condition, and water retention. In the long term, the symptoms come and go in waves so that the energy is up and down, but "never as it was before." Sometimes the condition can be explained as "never well after a heavy flu," or "tired since glandular fever," even "tired of being tired." These symptoms can be combined with many others depending on the different organs affected.

EAV test for viruses

The EAV test for viruses is possible by using specific testers that are homeopathic nosodes for different viral pathogens. They can be prepared by the usual homeopathic procedure of trituration of powders or solution and potentization of liquids based on material containing viral antigens or antibodies produced against the pathogen, or by electronic devices, charging the specific electromagnetic frequency onto milk sugar, distilled water, or alcohol solution. These substances are capable of storing the information in their structure. The EAV test for viruses is based on the measurements of three meridians: Al–Immune System (Right and Left), Ly–Lymphatic System (Right and Left), and RP/SP–Spleen (Left). In addition, MC-9/CI-7b can be tested. This is the point of the lymphatic system in the meridian of the circulation. This point can be an indicator for toxins in the lymphatic system and often is a signal for water retention.

Often normal signals from the right side of the first two meridians (Al, Ly) can be seen, but high signals appear on the left side. It is most important to test the spleen. The signals from the points RP-1/SP-1 and RP-4/SR-2 are connected with the production of white blood cells. A high signal is an indicator for some inflammation. The other points of the meridian RP are sensitive as well. In some cases of chronic viral infection, high signals from each of the points of the meridian of the spleen can be seen. The point MC-9/CI-7b often shows a high signal, which is worse on the left side. This is an indicator of loading of the lymphatic system with toxins. The patients with chronic viral infection often have edema of the lower extremities and sometimes generalized water retention. The spleen can be affected for other reasons such as diseases of the blood, or bacterial, fungal, or parasitic infections. Testing for the last three is necessary. After discovering the viral pathogen, the next step should be the testing of the meridians of organs and systems affected by the virus. After that a test for the combination of remedy and natural supplements is necessary.

The natural treatment of viruses

The treatment of viruses in the natural way includes homeopathic medications and an immune booster. The homeopathic treatment of chronic viral infections includes a homeopathic nosode and a homeopathic remedy.

It is important to support the immune system with immune boosters, mainly antioxidants. The best vitamins for viral infections are Vitamins A, C, and E. Usually it is necessary to have three to six months of intensive homeopathic treatment before the spleen returns to normal; in some heavy viral infections, even eight months is required. After the signal from the spleen becomes normal, it is advisable to repeat the homeopathic remedy for another month. It is also advisable to change the remedy after one or two months.

Homeopathic remedies for viral infections, confirmed by Voll testing

The main homeopathic remedies, which we found by Voll testing, for chronic viral infections are the MERCURY SALTS: Mercurius solubilis, Mercurius vivus, Mercurius iodatus flavus, Mercurius dulcis, Mercurius iodatus rubber, Mercurius phosphoricum, and Cinnabaris, in different potencies from 6 CH to 200 CH. Higher potencies are rarely required. Other groups of homeopathic remedies, confirmed by Voll tests, which produce beneficial effects for viral infections, include: Argentum metallicum, Antimonium crudum, Arsenicum iodatum, Carbo animalis, Carbo vegetabilis, Carboneum sulphuratum, Chelidonium, China, Chininum arsenicum, Chininum sulphuricum, Colchicum, Cuprum metallicum, Gelsemium, Glonoinum, Hydrastis Canadensis, Kalium arsenicosum, Lathyrus, Natrium arsenicosum, Nux vomica, Phosphorus, Sulphur, and Teucrium.

Usupov confirmed by Voll testing the following remedies:

Baryta carbonica for adenoviruses; Causticum and Rhus tox for CMV; Cardius marianus for Hepatitis, and a number of remedies for Herpes virus: Arsenicum album, Acidum muriaticum, Bufo rana, Causticum, Clematis, Croton tigrinum, Digitalis, Dulcamara, Hepar sulphuricum, Kreosotum, Natrium muriaticum, Petroleum, Psorinum, Rhus toxicodendron, Sepia, Strophanthus, Sulphur, Tellurium, and Thuja [Usupov, 2000]. The homeopathic remedies for viral infections found by the Voll test are presented in Table 5. It is essential that these remedies be tested on the meridian points of the spleen. Even for members of the same family diagnosed with the same virus, each individual needs a different homeopathic remedy in a different potency. Substances for boosting the immune system should be prescribed stringently, they should also be tested.

Vitamin C and antioxidants must be taken for this condition. According to the general condition and the results of the tests on the meridians of the organs and systems, individual measures for supporting the organs should be taken.

5.3.4.1. EPSTEIN–BARR VIRUS (EBV)

Epstein–Barr virus belongs to the group of herpes viruses. The virus is one of the most common of our time. It can be spread by contact with infected saliva or blood transfusion. Often it can be contracted in schools, military camps, shopping centers, or in airbuses. EBV was first found in tumors of Burkitt's lymphoma. It can be found in lymphoblasts of individuals with infectious mononucleosis, but also in visibly healthy individuals. Antibodies persist at a reduced level for many years. Laboratory confirmations of the presence of EBV in the blood of individuals with Burkitt's lymphoma, Hodgkin's disease, Chronic lymphatic leukaemia, and Sarcoidosis are often found, but the role of EBV in these conditions is not clear. The virus attacks B- and T-lymphocytes. The blood tests for EBV are not completely reliable [Mackie & McCartney, 1978]. Through the experience and complaints of many sufferers, EBV infection can be described by the following symptoms:

Epstein–Barr virus infection, the main symptoms

- People are tired, sleepy, exhausted, forcing themselves to do their daily obligations with difficulty
- Flu-like symptoms, long-lasting periods of viral infection
- Fever periodically, hot flushes, perspiration
- Dizzy, bilious, with vertigo and nausea
- Anemia
- Hormonal imbalances, including adrenal, reproductive, and thyroid glands
- Inflamed lymphatic glands periodically and over a long time
- Numbness of the feet, sore feet, swollen feet
- Anxiety, depression, panic attacks
- Headaches often that are severe
- Memory and concentration problems

Sometimes only one or two symptoms are manifested, and tiredness is the most prominent.

Homeopathic remedies for Epstein–Barr virus infection, confirmed by Voll testing

Through Voll testing we found many homeopathic remedies that are useful for EBV: Mercury salts such as Cinnabaris, Mercurius iodatus rubber, Mercurius dulcis, Mercurius solubilis, Mercurius vivus; other salts such as Antimonium crudum, Arsenicum iodatum, Chininum arsenicosum, Glonoinum, Kalium arsenicosum, and Natrium arsenicosum (Table 5). Vitamin C is useful, too; through Voll testing it was found that many other antioxidants are also beneficial, as they neutralize the toxins from the viruses. Immune boosters and immune modulators are important. There are many of them on the market. For each client the necessary supplements are different. Testing on the points of the spleen is essential. Every month or two the action of the remedy has to be tested again, and usually then it is replaced with something else, so as not to allow the virus to get used to the treatment.

5.3.4.2. COXSACKIE VIRUSES

Coxsackie viruses belong to the group of Enteroviruses. There are about thirty types in two big groups of Coxsackie viruses:

Group A comprises 24 types. They can cause severe myositis of the skeletal muscles, meningitis (types 2,4,7,9,23), mild paralysis (type 7), hand, foot, and mouth disease (types 5,16), and respiratory problems (type 21).

Group B comprises 6 types. They can cause myositis, tremors, incoordination, paralysis (spastic type), meningoencephalitis, pancreatitis, Epidemic myalgia (Bornholm disease with stitching pain in the muscles of the chest and epigastrium), myocarditis and pericarditis in newborn infants (types 2,3,4,5), skin rashes (types 1,3,5), and herpangina. Practically every organ can be infected by these viruses. The infection comes through the oral–fecal route. The virus isolation and serological blood tests are burdensome, but useful for the diagnosis. EAV testing can be done if testers, i.e. nosodes for the pathogens, are available. If the specific nosode is available for Coxsackie virus as a group and for differentiation of the types in the group,

166

the test is quick and does not need the use of blood samples or chemicals.

Coxsackie virus symptoms

From a practical point of view the main complaints and symptoms can be described as follows:

- muscle pain, especially neck and chest pain
- joint pain
- swollen glands
- weakness, sleepiness, tiredness
- migraines and headaches, sometimes with dizziness and vomiting
- sore throat, spasms of the throat
- anemia
- pain in the area of the heart, problems of the valves of the heart
- fever and perspiration at night
- swollen legs, water retention
- irregular menses, pain in the ovaries
- skin rashes
- difficult concentration, learning problems, epileptic fits
- flu and colds are often contracted

Homeopathic remedies for Coxsackie virus infection, confirmed by Voll testing

The homeopathic remedies for Coxsackie viruses include Aurum sulphuricum, Hydrastis canadensis, and the group of Mercury salts: Cinnabaris, Mercurius corrosivus, Mercurius cyanatus, Mercurius iodatus flavus, Mercurius iodatus rubber, Mercurius solubilis, and Mercurius vivus (Table 5). The treatment includes a homeopathic nosode, homeopathic remedy, Vitamin C, antioxidants, and immune boosters. The treatment lasts three to six months with the changing of the homeopathic remedy every one or two months. When the spleen reaches a normal signal, then the last combination of medicine is repeated for one more month. Later, after three months, it is advisable to do the test for the virus again. Typical examples of cases of Coxsackie Virus are described in Chapter Six: Case Studies.

5.3.4.3. CYTOMEGALO VIRUS (CMV)

Cytomegalo virus belongs to the herpes group of viruses. The infected blood cells become swollen (40 µm in diameter) with intracellular inclusions, which assists the laboratory diagnosis using a microscope. Blood tests for CMV are available, but patients have such a broad variety of symptoms that often the diagnosis of this viral infection is missed. The majority of the clinical syndromes are unrecognized. The virus can be found in urine and saliva, so the infection is relatively easily contracted in public places. A serious source can be blood transfusion. It is noted in the literature that the kidneys, liver, salivary glands, and spleen are often affected, and a persistent enlargement of the liver and spleen can be observed. The virus can cause Hemolytic anemia, Myocarditis, Pericarditis, Polyneuritis, and Mononucleosis, and is a very serious condition for children. By EAV testing, numerous cases of CMV have been found, many of which had been left without a real diagnosis and proper treatment for years. Most often cases occur with symptoms of:

- tiredness, sleepiness, fatigue
- headaches for years
- depression, claustrophobia, panic attacks, heart symptoms
- epileptic fits
- anemia, not affected by iron medications
- children not growing well physically and mentally
- concentration problems
- children with cerebral palsy
- affected thyroid, adrenal, and pituitary glands
- disturbed function of the pancreas with low or high insulin level, or disorder of other pancreatic enzymes
- men with enlarged prostate glands
- women with problems of the ovaries, irregular and painful menstruation
- families with infertility and repeated miscarriages

Homeopathic remedies for Cytomegalo virus infection, confirmed by Voll testing

According to Usupov, good remedies for CMV found by Voll testing are Causticum and Rhus toxicodendron [Usupov, 2000]. With Voll testing we found a good response from the following remedies: Argentum metallicum, Ferrum iodatum, Teucrium, and Mercury salts such as Cinnabaris, Mercurius corrosivus, Mercurius cyanatus, Mercurius iodatus flavus, Mercurius iodatus ruber, Mercurius cyanatus, Mercurius solubilis, and Mercurius vivus (Table 5). The treatment of CMV includes a homeopathic nosode, homeopathic remedy, antioxidants, Vitamin C, and an immune booster. Everything is chosen after testing. Every one or two months a new test should be done and the medications changed. The treatment should continue for three to six months usually, and sometimes longer. Cases of CMV are presented in Chapter Six: Case Studies.

5.3.4.4. ROTAVIRUSES

Rotaviruses are known to cause diarrhea in infants and young children, called viral enteritis.

Six serological groups of Rotaviruses have been identified, and three of them (A, B, C) infect humans. The infection is through the oral–fecal route, by hands or contaminated water. The virus infects the lining of the intestine, mainly the cells of the intestinal villi, and it leads to impaired hydrolysis of carbohydrates and excessive loss of fluid from the intestine. The main problem is diarrhea with serious dehydration and weight loss in children. In adults symptoms usually include nausea, vomiting, low-grade fever, and cramping pain in the abdomen. Rotavirus excretions with lack of serious symptoms are not an exception for adults. The EAV test shows that very often the diarrhea in adults is not a significant symptom; Rotavirus can be diagnosed by the Voll test in the presence of common symptoms for viral infections. In spite of the opinion that extra-intestinal infection with Rotavirus can be seen only in immuno-compromised patients, our tests show that often not only the intestines but also other organs can be affected in non–immuno-compromised patients.

Homeopathic medicine for Rotaviruses

The homeopathic remedies for Rotaviruses are listed in Table 5 and they include: Carbo vegetabilis, Podophyllum, and Mercury salts. Vitamin C, antioxidants, and immune boosters are an important part of the treatment. A case of Rotavirus infection is described in Chapter Six: Case Studies.

5.3.4.5. HEPATITIS A–E AND G VIRUSES

Hepatitis is an inflammation of the liver. It is not a single disease. It can be caused by many different pathogens such as parasites, including protozoa and sporozoa, bacteria, viruses, or by the chemical influence of drugs and alcohol. A viral hepatitis can be caused by a variety of viruses: Rubella, Adenoviruses, Coxsackie viruses, Cytomegalo virus, Yellow fever virus, and Hepatitis A–E viruses. Hepatitis A–E viruses are the most common of the above causes of viral hepatitis. They seriously affect the function of the liver. Approximately 47% of cases are Hepatitis A virus, 34% are Hepatitis B virus, 16% are Hepatitis C virus, and 3% are other Hep viruses. The cause of 10–20% of acute A–E seronegative hepatitis cases remains unknown.

Hepatitis A virus (HAV)

Hepatitis A virus formerly was classified as Enterovirus. Later it was classified as a member of the family Picornaviruses. The size of the virus is 20–30 nm. The route of infection is oral–fecal, rarely by blood. There are cases of infection by consumption of shellfish. The incubation period is 10 to 50 days. The symptoms are usually fever, nausea, jaundice, dark urine and light stools, and pain in the limbs. Most of the childhood Hepatitis A infections and 25–50% of the adult infections are asymptomatic and atypical. The development of the infection includes raised levels of Immunoglobulin M (Ig M) in the blood. The increased level of Ig M appears 3–4 weeks after the contraction of the disease, persists for about 4 weeks, and after that disappears. The period of 4 weeks is the time in which a positive blood serological test will show. It corresponds to the acute phase of the infection. In chronic carriers, Immunoglobulin M is nonexistent in blood [Mackie & McCartney, 1978]. In most of the cases (99%), it is common to recover completely over several weeks; only a few cases experience permanent liver damage. There is a vaccine against Hepatitis A virus. Hepatitis A is one of the major uncontrolled infections of our time.

Hepatitis B virus (HBV)

Hepatitis B virus is the prototype member of the family Hepadnaviridae. The particles are spherical, 42–47 nm in diameter with a tubular tail. The infection can be transmitted by blood transfusion, dialysis, sexual contact (saliva and semen), trans-placental, and from breast milk.

Only humans and chimpanzees are susceptible to infection with HBV. The incubation period is 40 to 120 days. The infection develops slowly and Immunoglobulin M (Ig M) is rarely raised. Laboratory tests show a positive Australian antigen. Fever is rare, the symptoms are similar to those of HAV, but not acute, and slowly lead to chronic damage of the liver. More often than not HBV infection is in a chronic form. In tropical countries 5–10% of a "healthy" population with liver complaints have HBV. HBV may be carried in the blood for many years, even lifelong. This virus is connected with polyarteritis nodosa, systemic lupus erythematosus, and arthritis, but the most serious effect is on the liver where the virus can cause hepatocellular complications such as cirrhosis and hepatoma. There is a vaccine for HBV. For treatment, medicine such as Alpha-interferon, Peginterferon, Lamivudine, Adefovir, and Dipivoxil are available.

Hepatitis C virus (HCV)

Hepatitis C virus was identified in 1989, first placed in the family Flaviviridae and lately has been put in a new monotypic genus, Hepacivirus, in this family. It is estimated that about 90% of non-A non-B hepatitis is caused by the Hepatitis C virus. Six main types of HCV have been isolated worldwide, each with several subtypes. Types 1–3 account for almost all infections in Europe. Type 4 is in Egypt and Zaire. Type 5 is in South Africa. Type 6 is in Hong Kong. Hepatitis C virus is slow-acting like Hepatitis B, and the routes of infection are the same: by blood, sexual contact, trans-placental, and by breast milk. Hepatitis C virus is now the commonest cause of chronic cases of hepatitis and the increase is due to blood transfusion, transplants, and drug abuse. The virus cannot be cultured and so it is difficult to research its biology. There is no available vaccine for HCV. The medicine used for treatment is Peginterferon and Ribavirin. The risk of developing liver damage such as cirrhosis and cancer is similar to that of HBV.

Hepatitis D virus (HDV)

In 1977 Hepatitis D virus was discovered in the blood of patients with HBV Delta antigen. In 1980 it was demonstrated that HDV is a defective transmissible pathogen depending on HBV for its replication. There is evidence that the presence of HDV potentates the pathogenic effects of Hepatitis B virus. The treatment is with Alpha-interferon.

Hepatitis E virus (HEV)

In the most recent classification, HEV has been placed in its own taxonomic group within the class RNA viruses "Hepatitis E-like viruses." HEV is a particle 30–32 nm in diameter. Four different genotypes have been detected. The infection is transmitted through the oral–fecal (waterborne) route, as with Hepatitis A virus. The incubation period is one month. The infection is acute, but relatively benign, except in pregnant women. Serological (antibody-based) assays recently became available. Recombinant vaccines are currently being prepared.

Hepatitis G virus (GBV/HGV)

Hepatitis G virus was found in 1967 and was named GB-agent, but now it is known that there are A, B, and C types of it. It causes a self-limiting infection, similar to that of HBV. Subclinical infections are common, and 1–2% of blood donors test positive for HGV. The majority of patients infected do not develop chronic hepatitis, but viremia frequently persists without biochemical evidence.

EAV testing for Hepatitis viruses

The first signs of the presence of Hepatitis viruses is the EAV reading from the immune and lymphatic systems (Al, Ly). The liver gives a high reading (especially the points F-1,2,3/LV-1,1a,1b). The meridian of the spleen (RP/SP) is irritated, more or less depending on the condition. The EAV test is sensitive: It can detect the presence of the virus not only in the period of the increased antibodies Ig M, corresponding to an acute form of the hepatitis, but before and after their rise. So in some cases the serological blood test for the virus can be negative. This corresponds to a condition called *occult disease* or *hidden disease*. The virus is there, but the energy of the body and the internal environment are strong enough to prevent the development of the pathogen. If for some reason the energy level of the system drops, the barrier of prevention is broken and the virus will start to multiply. So, by EAV test, detecting the pathogen is easy, and this allows us to take timely measures for its inactivation and for boosting the energy of the body. This is the best action to take, as it is preventative medicine. This is the future of any medicine. Working like this, we are at risk of being misunderstood. We have to teach people to understand what happens within their bodies and that it is their own health and they are responsible for it. Our task is to help them with our knowledge, but the main work is done by the individual and by Nature. When the person is aware of the process of healing, they are supportive of their own health and the best results are achieved.

Homeopathic medicine for Hepatitis

In the R. Murphy Repertory many good remedies for Hepatitis are given [Murphy, 1996]: p. 415, Hepatitis, Acute—Aconite, Belladonna, Kalium carbonicum, Podophyllum, Sulphur; sub-acute—Chamomilla, Hydrastis; chronic—Arnica, Aurum metallicum, Belladonna, Carcinosinum, Carduus marianus, Cornus circinata, Crotalus horridus, Lachesis, Lycopodium, Magnesium muriaticum, Natrium carbonicum, Natrium muriaticum, Natrium sulphuricum, Nitricum acidum, Nux vomica, Phosphorus, psorinum, Ranunculus sceleratus, Selenium, Silicea, and Sulphur.

Homeopathic remedies for Hepatitis viral infection confirmed by Voll testing

According to Usupov, the remedy Carduus marianus is the best [Usupov, 2000]. Our Voll tests show that the following remedies work very well: Carbo animalis, Carbo vegetabilis, Carboneum sulphuratum, Chelidonium, China, Chininum arsenicosum, Chininum sulphuricum, Hydrastis Canadensis, Mercurius corrosivus, Mercurius cyanatus, Mercurius solubilis, and Nux vomica (Table 5). Excellent results are achieved from the combination of a homeopathic remedy with Vitamin C, antioxidants, and herbal supplements for the liver. However, everything has to be tested by the Voll machine before prescribing the remedy.

173

5.3.5. EAV AND HOMEOPATHY FOR FUNCTIONAL DISORDERS OF ORGANS AND SYSTEMS

The imbalance of energy in the human biological system is not simply caused by the invasion of pathogens. The pathogens survive only if the system permits them to live and to multiply in our bodies. Conditions for this situation can exist for a long time internally, causing a deformation of the energy field of the body. Sometimes without any invasion, the organs can be functionally out of their normal alignment. The EAV test can detect functional disorders very early, months, sometimes one or two years, before any clinical symptoms or laboratory biochemical evidence appears. Very often the patient feels that "something is wrong" or "it is not as before" or "never well since." The homeopaths know and listen carefully to this kind of information. Disorder of the internal biochemical and biophysical condition can be produced as a result of many factors.

A large part of our health problems are stress-related. The presence of long-lasting stress, unresolved emotional problems, or a situation where the person feels trapped and cannot "see the light at the end of the tunnel" can unlock a variety of problems on a physical level. Many seriously ill people explain that for a long time before their illness they had serious family or business problems, or persistent stress and negative emotions. Everybody has a weak spot in the body, and the problems start there. The same emotional situation can cause for one person a hormonal disorder, for another stomach pain or diabetes. That is why it is advisable before the EAV test to ask the patient about emotional problems. There are thousands of different problems, but the basic three groups are fears, anxiety, and illusions. Peter Chappell, a Vice Director of the London College of Classical Homeopathy, said in 1995, during one of his lectures on *Homeopathic Materia Medica* in Sofia, Bulgaria:

"We live in a prison named ego and its walls are our illusions and our fears. If we get over the ego, the whole world will be open to us. Materia Medica *studies the types of human ego and teaches us how to achieve freedom."*

The knowledge of homeopathic remedies, in the *Materia Medica*, especially the Mind section, is a great advantage to everyone doing EAV tests. Sometimes only one remedy is required to rebalance the whole meridian system of the patient. But is there any meridian point which can be used for testing emotions?

I know only one point for testing emotions. According to Chinese traditional medicine, the heart rules the emotions and the psychological function of man. The first point on the left side of the heart meridian (C-1/HE-9, left) at the physical level corresponds to the aortic valve. My experience revealed that this point is very sensitive to emotions and that it is useful for testing homeopathic remedies for emotional conditions. Perhaps some other more sensitive points can be found on this meridian. An experiment for testing constitutional remedies on the emotional point C-1/HE-9 or some other points should be done in future research. Some EAV practitioners use Bach flower remedies or herbal preparations for emotional conditions. They can be tested on the point C-1/HE-9 as well.

Malnutrition is another important cause of the dysfunction of the organs and systems. There are many countries in the world where food is a big problem and actual physical survival is sometimes in question. Surprisingly, malnutrition can be a problem in rich societies as well. Very often the quality of food supplied to the market is not what it should be. The fruit and vegetables are picked unripe and they are kept for a long time in refrigerators. Often they have uncontrolled amounts of nitrates and other fertilizers and as a result have lost their vitamins and minerals before reaching the consumer. Meat and chicken may be full of antibiotics and artificial hormones and these substances can disturb our physiology adversely. Preservatives and colorants could be a source of toxins in the body.

Toxins and chemicals can enter through heavy allopathic medications and uncontrolled use of supplements over a long time. Some people cannot imagine how to live healthfully without a handful of vitamins, minerals, and different hormonal and herbal supplements every day. They think that these are all natural and so harmless. I sometimes test supplements for my clients, who often have a big basket full of them. Usually only half of them or even fewer are any good for the client. Sometimes the combination of all of them shows a negative influence on some organs such as the liver and kidneys. Very often the best thing for the patient is to stop everything for a month.

The other source of disturbance of the energy of the organs is lack of oxygen. Lots of people live in big cities, with air polluted with industrial gases and petrol fumes, and they experience a permanent insufficiency of oxygen. Sedentary work and limited physical exercise are very common in civilized life. Increased anaerobic bacterial flora such as Clostridium difficile is a very common condition among people with digestive problems. It shows that the processes of oxidization are not efficient. If people with decreased oxygen take in additional antioxidants, it becomes even worse. That is why it is best to test all the supplements and to give advice on an individual basis. A good idea is to test oxidants and antioxidants to see what really works for that particular individual.

A lot is written about heavy metals in the body. Here I will mention only that there is evidence of a relationship between a chronic infestation of Candida and the presence of metal tooth fillings. Testing for heavy metals and suggesting cleaning procedures is a good way of improving health.

Increased acidity of the system is another very important cause of the disturbance of the normal function of the organs. According to Enderlein, this is the most serious cause of the development of microscopic parasitic proteins to higher more pathogenic stages in the blood. The pH test of saliva and urine is easy. If the test shows pH < 5 it means high acidity, and then the best thing to do is to alkalize the body. There are different alkalizing mixtures on the market.

Increased acidity of the body can be detected at point RP-4/SP-2 on the meridian of the pancreas, right side. A high reading shows uric acid diathesis. It usually indicates poor digestion of proteins, or that there are too many proteins in the diet.

Disorders of the hormonal system are very prevalent. More than 30% of clients suffer from a hormonal imbalance, though they do not realize it. Very often a person on chronic antidepressants simply needs to balance their hormones. Women on hormone replacement therapy often live in a condition of hormone imbalance, and they do not know why they are so nervous and aggressive.

One of the best scientifically developed parts of medicine is Endocrinology. It is a good strategy to replace material hormonal medicine with homeopathic nosodes for hormones. These are without side effects and rebalance the system. The EAV test is carried out on eight points of the meridian of the hormones TR/TW and two points of the meridian Urinary bladder: V-7/UB-65 and V-8/UB-64 (uterus and ovaries for women; prostate gland and testicles for men). Many natural supplements for hormones are on the market now, and if their application is confirmed by EAV test for a particular individual, they do work well.

I do not intend to explain how to test different organs, neither to suggest homeopathic remedies for organs. In this field, broad research on *Homeopathic Materia Medica* and on the *Repertories* should be done, but this is not the object of this book. I hope that some homeopaths will continue with research in the field of homeopathy using physical tests. This would be my reward for this pilot research.

The following Chapter 6: Case Studies will show some cases of detecting and treating different conditions by EAV. I hope that the reader will see the beauty of the method and will be convinced that the combination of EAV and homeopathy opens new horizons for homeopathy and for medicine.

CHAPTER 6

CASE STUDIES

Case 1 (4208-3-32) (Tuberculosis)

Nagao (age 42) had a febrile condition for six months. He was diagnosed with tuberculosis. He was treated with six different antibiotics, but none of them really improved his condition. At the time of his first visit in January 2002, he was yet again on an antibiotic. An EAV test found two types of pathogens: Streptococcus viridans and Mycobacterium bovinum. Positive signals from the meridians of the immune system (Al) and both lungs (P, LU) were found with the tester Tuberculinum bovinum 30 CH. A signal for Streptococcus in the sinuses was noticed. During the consultation he mentioned that every morning he drank fresh milk, not boiled, which was probably the source of the infection. The combination of the two nosodes for the pathogens and Mercurius corrosivus 12 CH was sufficient to return the meridians to the normal condition.

Rx: Tuberculinum bovinum 30 CH, Streptococcus 200 CH, Mercurius corrosivus 12 CH, and Royal jelly, a supplement for the immune system, made from bee products.

Because of the seriousness of the situation, it was suggested that the client have resonance vibration treatment by Driver Resonator machine of 365 KHz and 432 KHz every day. These frequencies correspond to the resonance vibrations of the pathogens found. Usually 10 sessions are recommended, 15 min on each frequency every day. He did 30 sessions of resonance vibrations in one month, and he took his remedies regularly.

After one month, in March 2002, the EAV test was negative for the two bacteria. The cough and the temperature had subsided. Two months later in May 2002 he came for a followup test and everything was normal. He felt very well, and really healthy the following year.

Case 2 (6483-5-173) (Mycoplasma pneumonia)

Four months previously, Abby (68) was diagnosed by means of a blood test as having Mycoplasma. During that period she was treated with three types of antibiotics and after that cortisone was prescribed. However, she continued coughing with bloody expectoration. She really did not feel well: her ears were blocked, her throat was sore, her sinuses were inflamed, and blood could be seen in the mucus. At the end of April 2003 she was tested by EAV. Two pathogens were detected: Streptococcus hemolyticus and Mycoplasma pneumonia. The signals came from the immune system, lymphatic system, lungs, liver, gallbladder, and spleen. The combination of the natural medicines recommended for normalizing the balance of the meridians is given below.

Rx: Streptococcus 30 CH, Mycoplasma 30 CH, Arsenicum album 200 CH, and Echinaforce drops for her immune system.

Two months later she came back looking very healthy. The cough had subsided, she felt very well, and all symptoms were cleared. The EAV test showed that the condition of all the organs was normal. The following two years she was clear.

Case 3 (6384-5-142) (Klebsiella)

Virginia (46) had a dry cough during the day for five months. She tried different cough syrups and antibiotics but nothing would alleviate the cough. She found a partial solution by taking honey and water in small sips often. The cough was accompanied by constant tightness of the chest. In March 2003 she was tested by EAV, and Klebsiella pneumonia was found, affecting the immune and lymphatic system, her left lung, and her liver. The following natural medicines in combination were necessary for normalizing the balance of the meridians.

Rx: Arsenicum album 30 CH, Klebsiella 30 CH, Iodum 200 CH (for the liver), and Propolis tablets.

The food allergy test showed that it was essential for her to completely stop taking sugar, crystal fructose, and dairy products. Fresh fruit was allowed, except for grapes, bananas, and watermelon.

Two months later, in May 2003, she reported that the cough had stopped quite quickly, that is only a week after starting taking the remedies.

A month later she had flu, but the cough was not the same as before and lasted only a week. Objectively the signal for Klebsiella was gone, according to the EAV test. The food test was repeated, and it was found that there was no need for the special diet anymore.

Case 4 (3042-2-163) (Staphylococcus)

Laura (40) had boils all over her body for more than a year. Every month about ten new boils would appear on different parts of her body. She was tired and often had headaches. During the most recent month she had really bad headaches. She also experienced pain in her small joints in the evenings. She had good digestion, regular bowel movement, and normal blood pressure. Antibiotics were prescribed very often, but none of them solved her problem. In January 2001 the EAV test showed Staphylococcus aureus with signals from the immune system, lymphatic system, liver, and spleen. A mixed nosode for Staphylococcus bacteria, homeopathic remedy Mercurius corrosivus 12 CH, and Vitamin C were sufficient for balancing the meridian system.

Rx: Staphylococcus 30/200 CH (mix), Mercurius corrosivus 12 CH, nonacidic Vitamin C.

Intolerance to coffee and Coca-Cola was found by an allergy test.

One month later she was very much better. During that period she had only two new boils and they appeared after taking sweet drinks. This time an EAV test found only two abnormal points: Al-3 in the immune system and RP-3/SP-1b (left) in the spleen. The medicine was repeated. In November 2001 she reported that the boils had vanished completely in March (after three months of treatment) and they had never come back again.

Case 5 (579-1-21) (Streptococcus)

Matt (37) came for his first consultation in August 1998. He had repeated throat infections appearing with changes in the weather. He was coughing with white mucus mixed with red and yellow strings. He had to talk a lot and with many people as he was a merchant and he needed his throat to be strong and healthy. After many courses of different antibiotics, his problem still persisted. An EAV test revealed a Streptococcus infection. The most prominent signal was in the lymphatic system, on the point of the tonsils (Ly-1/Ly-1-1). The meridian Ly was balanced by the following combination of remedies.

Rx: Streptococcus 30 CH and Phosphorus 200 CH.

A month later the patient was in very good health, and he had no complaints about his throat and tonsils. The expectoration subsided. The EAV test showed only one slight signal from the meridian of the lymphatic system. He was under huge stress, because his wife had had a miscarriage the previous week. After that he could not fall asleep, he used to lie in bed thinking. By testing the point C-1/He-9, a combination for calming his emotional condition was found.

Rx: Natrium arsenicum 30 CH, Staphysagria 200 CH.

In October he was absolutely clear and had no complaints about his throat. Subsequently he was very well, and his throat was no longer a problem for him.

Case 6 (2-132) (Malaria)

Orlando (37) in August 2000 had flu-like symptoms for three weeks, with perspiration at night and abdominal pain below his ribs on his sides and back. One year previously during the same period he had had Malaria, which was cured in the hospital. After that his liver was sensitive to alcohol and he often had pain in the stomach. An EAV test revealed signals for the Malaria plasmodium pathogen. His liver, pancreas, and spleen were very irritated. Malaria 30 CH nosode worked well to balance these three meridians. In addition, he had a signal from the duodenum, which responded to Helicobacter pylori 3CH. The best combination of remedies for normalizing his meridian system was the following.

Rx: Malaria 30 CH, Helicobacter pylori 3 CH, and Bismutum subnitricum 6 CH.

Two months later he explained that after taking the remedies for one month he felt well. He then stopped the remedies for one week, but the night sweats started again. The medications were repeated for one more month and he felt very well. The symptoms of Malaria vanished and the stomach pain also disappeared. An EAV test showed a normal reading for the tested organs: liver, spleen, pancreas, and stomach. The recommended remedies were repeated for another month. It was suggested he take lemon and honey in water, twice a day. After the treatment, he had no signals or symptoms of Malaria anymore.

Case 7 (2755-2-130) (Fasciolopsis buscii)

Pamela (51) came in during September 2000 and was diagnosed with cysts in the liver and kidney. She had had two other diagnoses before this, spastic colon and hiatus hernia, but lately she experienced pain in different parts of her body: dull pain in the lower back, pain in the epigastrium and in the upper abdomen on both sides. Because of these persistent pains she was sent for computer tomography to scan her internal organs, and as a result lots of cysts were found: four cysts in the liver and one in the left kidney. It was suggested to her that she should wait and observe the development of the cysts. After one month the cysts in the liver grew bigger. The opinion of the doctor was that an operation was impossible. An EAV test revealed a picture of infestation with the fluke Fasciolopsis buskii with signals from the liver, spleen, gallbladder, and left kidney. The treatment was with herbal preparations.

Rx: Paragon tincture and PARA-90 capsules.

She had vibrational treatment with a Driver Resonator machine (33 KHz and the specific vibration for Fasciolopsis of 432 KHz) twice a day for 21 days, and the signals for Fasciolopsis disappeared from the organs.

A second scanning of the liver four months after the treatment showed the cysts were in small pieces. EAV tests five and seven months later revealed a normal condition for the organs. The last test was done four years later, in July 2004. She was very well, and only the fear of future pain in the abdomen made her come in for tests.

Case 8 (6140-5-168) (Schistosoma, or Bilharzia)

Joyce (16) was not well for more than four years. She had a very pale, yellow complexion. She was often very tired, always hungry, with concentration problems at school and allergic reactions to many vitamins and medications. Her mother was very anxious about her health, sure that something was not right in spite of other opinions. In November 2002 the EAV test found signals for Bilharzia coming from her immune system (point Al-3), her liver (F/LV), spleen (RP/SP), and gallbladder (VB/GB). These meridians went to normal status after using the following combination.

183

Rx: Bilharzia 30 CH, Paragon tincture.

One month later the liver and the spleen were clear, point Al-3 was normal; still, the gallbladder gave a signal for a slight irritation. By testing on the meridian of the gallbladder (VB), a suitable remedy was found.

Rx: Acidum picricum 30 CH.

In February 2003, three months later, her liver was not well because she had taken some supplement for the immune system, on the advice of a friend. She ended up in the hospital with an allergic reaction and an asthma attack. She had no signs of parasites, but she needed a cleansing of the liver. By testing the meridian (F), one remedy was recommended.

Rx: Nux vomica 200 CH.

After six months, in June 2003, I saw her for the last time. The test for Bilharzia was negative, she was very well, with a nice, rosy complexion, happy and healthy.

Case 9 (2743-2-140) (Ascaris worms)

Damon (52) was a businessman with a very stressful life. He had severe diarrhea for a long time with a fever, and eventually he went to the hospital. After a colonoscopy, he was diagnosed with Crohn's disease. He was prescribed an anti-inflammation medicine, and it was suggested he take Cortisone. In September 2000 he was tested by EAV, which showed a severe infestation of Ascaris worms. The EAV signals were detected in meridians of the immune system (Al) and bowels (GI/LI and IG/SI).

Rx: Vermox 500 mg (a single dose), continuing with PARA-90 capsules for four weeks.

One month later the signal for the worms had disappeared. After that, at the end of October, he had another colonoscopy and there were no signs of Crohn's disease. His doctor asked him about what treatment he had had, and he replied that he took herbal medicine, but he never told the doctor about the worms.

Case 10 (4559-4-5) (Helicobacter pylori)

Mildred (54) had stomach complaints for years. She was diagnosed with gastritis of the stomach and IBS (Irritable Bowel Syndrome). She felt constantly bloated. Her chronic disorder of bowel movements was both diarrhea and constipation, often alternating, and she had pain in the left side of her colon. For years she took a number of laxatives and medications to control her digestion, but the relief was short-lived. In April 2002 the EAV test revealed irritation of the right side of the meridian of the immune system (Al-1,2,3) on the main point of the stomach (E-4/ST-44b) (which responded to Helicobacter pylori tester), a signal in the colon (GI/LI), and in addition she had a very irritated pancreas (RP/SP) and gallbladder (VB/GB). The Voll reading of these meridians went to normal when tested with Arsenicum iodatum 200 CH, which was recommended to be taken for one month.

Rx: Arsenicum iodatum 200 CH.

The allergy test described lots of foods that she could not tolerate: dairy products, alcohol, coffee, tea, cake flower, chlorinated water; different vegetables such as ginger, garlic, green beans; also some acidic fruits were not good for her such as pineapple, guava, grapes, kiwi fruit, and oranges. These foods were not allowed for three months. She was disciplined, she adhered to the diet, and she took her remedy regularly.

Within two months she felt very well, she felt practically healthy. The EAV test showed that her digestive system had returned to a normal condition. Everything was normal: stomach, colon, pancreas, gallbladder, and immune system. The homeopathic remedy was recommended for one more month. Eighteen months later at the beginning of November 2003 she reported that she was not taking any medicine. When she adhered to the diet, her digestive system stayed well.

Case 11 (6070-6-14) (E-coli in the urinary tract)

Randolph (48) had three main complaints when he came for Voll testing in October 2002: postnasal drip, lower back pain, and urination about twelve times during the night. He did not even complain but only mentioned that all his life he had had flatulence of the abdomen. He stopped taking sugar, sweets, and chocolate, and he lost six kilograms, but the frequent urination continued. An EAV test revealed signals for E-coli from the colon (GI /LI), both kidneys (R/KI), and the spleen (RP/SP). A food test showed that sugar, sweet fruits, and alcohol were the worst foods for him (sugar, honey, dried fruit, chocolate, grapes, sweet potatoes, sweet melon, pineapple, bananas, vinegar, wine, beer, and spirits). To balance the meridians, he needed a combination of the following natural medicines.

Rx: E-coli 30 CH, Cantharis 200 CH, and Acidophilus plus.

In December 2002 he reported that the frequent urination was much less but he still had the same lower back pain. He complained about a fungal infection on the skin of his right foot.

Objectively, the signals from E-coli had disappeared. After testing the meridian of the skin (S/SK), the following good combination of remedies for his fungus was found.

Rx: Acidum phosphoricum 200 CH, and Acidophillus plus.

For the lower back pain, a visit to a chiropractor was suggested.

Case 12 (6817-6-16) (Sycotic miasm)

According to Cedric (52), he was generally well. He was on medications for hypertension and for cholesterol and his condition was under control. From time to time he experienced gout pain in one of his toes. In addition he sometimes had pain from an old injury of the shoulder that had been operated on. He was very active, busy at work, with normal sleep and a normal digestion. In August 2003 the Voll test showed his left frontal sinus (Ly-6/Ly-3) was slightly inflamed, and a number of irritations (high signals) appeared from his immune system (Al), liver (F/LV), kidneys (R/KI), circulation (MC/CI), and pancreas and spleen (RP/SP). All these signals were improved when tested with the remedy Medorrhinum 30 CH. This remedy showed the presence of a sycosis in the system. I started explaining to him about this type of miasmatic influence, and he remembered that twenty years previously he had been infected and cured of gonorrhea.

Rx: Medorrhinum 30 CH and Cinnabaris 6 CH.

A food test was done and it was suggested that he reduce the intake of sugar, dairy products, red meat, pork meat, eggs, and vinegar.

At the end of October 2003, two months later, he reported that his sinus was well, he had lost one kilogram, the last blood test for cholesterol was normal, and his blood pressure was 136/80. He explained that he felt a dramatically improved mental sharpness. The Voll test showed that his organs were in normal condition and all signals were normal. It was suggested to him that he stay on the diet and repeat the remedies for a further month.

Case 13 (6030-6-7) (Asthma from Candida)

Sylvester (38) had been an asthma sufferer all his life, since he was a baby. He used to keep asthma inhalers in his pockets all the time, even near the swimming pool and when he was at the gym, because he suffered tightness of his chest from any exertion. At the time of his first visit in October 2002, he was using two inhalers, a bronchodilator and a steroid atomizer, once a day, sometimes more often. He felt that he put on weight easily. The Voll test revealed a signal for Candida albicans coming from his immune system (Al), lymphatic system (Ly), and both lungs (P /LU). The recommendation for him was the most common one for a yeast infestation, and it includes the nosode for Candida, natural antioxidants, and measures for restoring good flora in the gut.

Rx: Candida 30 CH, Antioxidant Proanthocyanidin, Vitamin C 1,000 mg, and Acidophilus.

He was put on a special diet which excluded dairy, sugar, and starch products (Table 2).

Two months later he was very well. He had been diligent with the diet and had lost four kilograms. He realized that he could run more easily and he did not need his inhalers lately. A Voll test showed normal signals from his lungs (P/LU) and immune and lymphatic systems (Al, Ly). The combination of remedies was recommended for a further month. Eight months later his lungs, lymphatic, and immune system were tested again and were normal. He reported that he did strenuous exercise and did not need an inhaler during that time. He had no symptoms of asthma anymore. One year later he visited me together with his wife, and when I asked him "How is the asthma?" his answer was: "No asthma at all."

Case 14 (6568-6-14 A) (Hepatitis A)

Beverly (57) felt very weak and nauseous for two weeks. A rash appeared on her chest. Before this she had had flu-like symptoms which changed to nausea and dizziness. Lately she could not get out of bed in the morning. She developed a very yellow complexion and she always felt exhausted. On May 28, 2003, her blood test confirmed Hepatitis A, and her doctor suggested resting and vegetarian food but she had no appetite at all. She had no medications for Hepatitis. The next day an EAV test found signals from the immune and lymphatic systems (Al, Ly), liver (F/LV), and spleen (RP/SP), which responded to the tester for Hepatitis A. She needed the following combination of natural medicine to normalize the reading from her meridians.

Rx: Hepatitis (mixed nosode) 30 CH, Chininum arsenicum 200 CH, nonacidic Vitamin C, and Coenzyme Q-10.

This combination rebalanced her system.

Two months later, in July 2003, she was very happy and she said that she had never been so well. The only thing that reminded her of Hepatitis was the fact that she could not take rich food. Rich food made her feel heavy and her eyes became red. The EAV test revealed a normal reading for her immune system, liver, and spleen. The remedies were repeated once more. The last EAV test was done after another three months, in October 2003. She had a cold and cough, she complained of menopausal hot flushes, but the Voll test for Hepatitis was negative.

Case 15 (6364-5-183) (Clostridium difficile)

Jake (67) had digestive problems for six years with loose stools and indigestion. He was sure that milk aggravated his condition and that chocolate caused him bad headaches. Often he did not sleep well and he knew that in the morning he would have diarrhea. From time to time he experienced joint pain in the left foot and the fingers of the right hand. His eyes were constantly red. In January 2003 the Voll test gave a normal reading for his organs: liver, pancreas, spleen, lungs, kidneys, and bladder. Signals of irritation appeared from his immune and lymphatic system (Al, Ly), intestines (GI/LI, IG/SI), and gallbladder (VB/GB) which corresponded to Clostridium difficile bacterium. The remedy which balanced these meridians was Bryonia alba 30 CH.

Rx: Clostridium difficile 30 CH and Bryonia alba 30 CH.

It was suggested that he should keep his diet free of sugar, milk, cheese, and bread (Table 4).

After two months, in March 2003, he felt that his digestion was not good enough, and he was not happy with keeping to the diet. Objectively, his immune and lymphatic systems improved, but the intestines and the gallbladder were still irritated. I decided to increase the oxygen in his digestive system with the following.

Rx: Cellfood drops, Acidum phosphoricum 30 CH, and Clostridium diff. 30 CH.

In May 2003 he showed great improvement in his digestive system. For the first time in six years his stools had formed normally. Objectively, a Voll test showed that the gallbladder was clear. The intestines needed more attention.

Rx: Cellfood drops and Kalium bichromicum 12 CH.

In July 2003 he was even better: The stool was normal and well-formed, the joints were well, and pain had disappeared. Jake was very happy and thankful. The EAV test showed a normal reading for all of his meridians. From the food test done, we noticed that there was no need for any diet now. I suggested to him that in the case of any future problems with his digestion, that it would be a good idea for him to go back to the diet.

Case 16 (1563-2-100) (A child with asthma and eczema)

Marcel (8) had had eczema and asthma since he was a baby. The skin of his arms, feet, and chest was badly affected: He had a very pale skin with very red spots of eczema with groups of small vesicles and yellow scales around them. The eczema got better or worse, but never cleared during these years. The child had a chronic sinus problem with postnasal drip. He used to cough a lot, especially in the morning on waking. For the asthma, he was on a Ventolin inhaler every day. He was small for his age, not growing well, with a pale face and dark rings under his eyes. The worst allergens for him were bananas and eggs, according to his mother. During his first visit to me in September 1999, a Voll test showed many irritated points on the meridian of the immune and lymphatic systems (Al, Ly), lungs (P/LU), and skin (S/SK). Allergy testing showed many other allergens: dairy products, peanuts, rye, oats, rice, wheat, broccoli, carrots, peaches, cucumbers, garlic, tomatoes, oranges, tea, feathers, and house dust. The child was advised to avoid those foods for at least three months. The following combination balanced his meridians.

Rx: Kalium bichromicum 6 CH, Sabadilla 200 CH, Mixed pollens 30 CH, and vitamins for children.

Two months later in November 1999 the child came to me with a dramatic improvement: He had no cough, the eczema had vanished, the asthma had subsided, and the atomizer had not been used lately. The dark rings under his eyes had disappeared. His mother said that he had much more energy and that he was a happy child now. The Voll test showed normal readings for the meridians. In December 1999 and in February 2000 the child came for testing and everything was fine. The last control test was one year later in May 2001, when the child was very well.

Case 17 (1185-2-60) (A very allergic child)

Ali (5) was a very allergic child. He often suffered from tonsilitis, sore ears, respiratory tract infections, and pain above the eyes. At the first visit in April 1999, he had a thick discharge from his nose of a white–yellow color and he was coughing a lot. His mother explained that the child had had these problems since the family moved to Johannesburg. The child had been tested for allergies by a blood test and two allergens had been found: eggs and dairy products. These foods were avoided but the allergy continued. The Voll allergy test revealed 32 allergens. Among them were wheat, sugar, fructose, oats, chicken, garlic, grass, dog hair, chlorine, house dust, feathers, and aspirin. According to our protocols the allergens should be avoided for three months. The immune and lymphatic systems (Al, Ly) were very irritated, but the meridians of the organs were in good condition. To balance the meridians it was necessary to give histamine in a homeopathic form.

Rx: Kalium muriaticum 6 CH and Sinu-histaplex homeopathic drops.

One month later in May 1999 the child still had a blocked nose in the morning and a runny nose during the day. The cough was much better and he coughed only occasionally. This time the histamine drops were not necessary.

Rx: Kalium muriaticum 6 CH, Phosphorus 200 CH, and Allergy formula drops.

In June 1999 the child had much more energy, the cough stopped completely, and the discharges from the nose were much less and quite clear. The EAV test still showed an irritated immune system, but a much-improved lymphatic system. The allergy test was repeated and we found only two allergens: sugar and dog hair.

Rx: Sambucus homeopathic drops.

In July the immune system was normal. The mother reported that during the last month the child was very well with no cough and no mucus from the nose. They came for a test, because the previous evening about 9 p.m. the child had had a little cough and a little bit of clear mucus. The allergy test showed no allergens. We recommended the following.

Rx: Pulsatilla 200 CH and Rose hips herbal tea.

This is a case that is typical of children with allergies. In children it is possible to clear the allergy in 3–4 months. After the age of 20 it is more difficult, but even some older people improve greatly if they adhere strictly to the diet.

Case 18 (1270-2-75) (Depression – hormonal imbalance)

Gladis (30) had had a baby in the previous year, and since that childbirth she had not been well. She was diagnosed with depression, anemia, and glandular fever. She had put on much weight lately, she was very tired and pale, she had water retention and was bloated. The menstrual cycle after the delivery was 24–25 days with severe premenstrual tension, previously it had been 28–35 days. She worked on a computer for long hours. On the first visit in May 1999, allergies to chicken, spinach, potatoes, peas, and coffee were found. The organs generally were healthy. Abnormal signals were found only from her spleen (RP/SP) and her hormonal system (TR/TW). The reading showed a hyperfunction of the adrenal glands and hypofunction of the thyroid gland, right side. A combination of two remedies balanced the meridians.

Rx: Phosphorus 200 CH and Thyreoidea 30 CH.

In June she was much better. Menstruation came on the 27th day. The hormonal meridian (TR/TW) and the meridian of the spleen (RP/SP) were normal. In July she was again tired and the cycle came on the 25th day. The following was the best combination for her hormonal meridian (TR/TW).

Rx: Folliculinum 15 CH, Lachesis 30 CH.

In November she was happy: No depression and no tiredness and she had lost 12 kg. The thyroid gland was balanced. The reading for the adrenal gland was still high. I have found that many remedies containing Natrium work well for this condition.

Rx: Natrium phosphoricum 6 CH.

After that she was well.

Case 19 (3480-2-180) (Salmonella)

Victoria (73) had a confirmed Salmonella infection from eating chicken meat ten months previously. She developed a red rash on the skin of her body and blue spots on her legs the size of coins. Since then the spots and the rash had remained, and new ones continued to appear with itchiness. She felt sick after taking food, even water in a large amount felt heavy in her stomach, so she had to take small sips of drinks often. The worst reaction for her was to sugar. Two hours after a meal she had a burning tongue and ringing ears. She felt so weak that sometimes she fainted. Her stool was very loose and on some days it became diarrhea. Recently she had been diagnosed with anemia. She lost weight until she was only 42 kg, weak, and skinny. On June 1, 2001, the Voll test found Salmonella bacteria in her bowels (GI/LI and IG/SI). The other affected organs were liver (F/LV), and pancreas and spleen (RP/SP). The meridian of the skin (S/SK) showed irritation. Among the many remedies I tested, the best for balancing the meridians was Arsenicum album 200 CH.

Rx: Arsenicum 200 CH (× 6 doses a day for 6 days, after that × 3 doses a day).

The food test showed sensitivity to sugar, milk, and starchy foods. She was advised to avoid these foods.

On June 18 she reported that her diarrhea had stopped, and she had even been constipated for two days. Still, she had a rash and itchy skin. On June 25, she had no diarrhea and no burning tongue anymore, the rash continued improving, and the itch subsided. After that she was well.

Case 20 (3080-5-176) (Chlamydia)

Jeffry (45) came to me in May 2003 with severe pain in his left knee. For two weeks the pain continued and physiotherapy did not help him. The Voll test found a Chlamydia infection. The affected meridians were liver (F/LV), spleen (RP/SP), left kidney (R/KI), and joints (Ad/JO). The best medication for balancing his meridians was the homeopathic remedy Argentum nitricum.

Rx: Chlamydia 30 CH and Argentum nitricum 30 CH.

The food test showed that wheat, alcohol, and vinegar had to be avoided. As the protocol required, he stopped these foods for three months.

After two months the signal for Chlamydia disappeared. The reading from the meridians was normal. The joint pain diminished. It was suggested that he take the remedies and continue the diet for one more month.

Case 21 (1837-2-112) (Candida, affecting kidneys)

Juanita (38) suffered from chronic fatigue for 18 years. She said that she was so tired that even "her heart does not want to beat." She was depressed, tense, anxious, and everything was too difficult for her, even her eyes were heavy and puffy with dark rings under them. She experienced dull pain in the abdomen and in the lower back. Her stools were not normal. She had alternating diarrhea and constipation. She realized that her digestion was better when she was on a protein diet. Previously she had been prescribed the homeopathic remedy Sepia, but without any improvement in her condition. In January 2000 she was tested by EAV. The organs generally were in a good condition, but a very high signal corresponding to Candida albicans came from her immune system (Al-1) and both kidneys (R/KI). The combination of bio-flora capsules, antioxidants, and a homeopathic nosode was the best remedy for balancing her meridian system.

Rx: Acidophilus plus, Carotene plus, nonacidic Vitamin C, Candida 30 CH.

She was put on a special diet excluding sugar, starch, dairy products, and alcohol (Table 4).

In February she was unbelievably well: no fatigue, no depression, no anxiety, no pain. Bowel movements had improved. She explained that she felt a reaction from the kidneys with dark, bad-smelling urine, and a feeling of soreness in the area for one week, and after that the urine became clear. Her sleep improved also. She now had plenty of energy and her eyes were not puffy anymore. The Voll test showed that Candida was still there, and the signals were still not normal. We had to continue the same medications and the diet. Usually three to four months are necessary to clear the yeast infection Candida. If the diet is not followed strictly, the problem can persist for more than six months. In March she arrived in a very good mood with good energy. The reading from the Voll test was normal. She was very well, but my suggestion was that she follow the diet and the remedies for one more month.

Case 22 (6258-5-163) (Rickettsia)

Anita (36) had felt depressed and tired for a while. She was a student at the university and she had difficulty concentrating. She had diarrhea often and generally bad digestion. For some reason her blood sugar level used to drop suddenly. Sometimes she had palpitations. She was diagnosed with Coxsackie virus in 1999 and cured by a homeopath. Now she wondered whether she had the virus again. In January 2003 she was tested by EAV. A strong signal for Rickettsia appeared from her immune system (Al, left side), lymphatic system (Ly, left side), liver (F/LV), and spleen (RP/SP, left side). The best combination of remedies to create a good balance in her meridians was the following.

Rx: Rickettsia mix 30 CH, Bellis perrenis 30 CH, Vitamin C 1,000 mg, Carotene plus, and Intestiflora.

A special diet was suggested: generally no wheat, sugar, milk, or alcohol (Table 4).

In March 2003 she was much better. Her concentration was better and she had more energy. She tried her best to keep to the diet. Objectively, her liver (F/LV) and her immune and lymphatic systems (Al, Ly) were normal. The signal for Rickettsia was detected only from the spleen (RP/SP, left). The diet and the medications were continued. She was tested again in June 2003. During the previous two months she had had exams with lots of stress but she was healthy all the time. The Voll test gave perfect results, her meridians had normal readings for everything tested. She was healthy in September 2003 when she came for the last test.

Case 23 (6124-5-30) (Chronic fatigue, Rickettsia)

Gina (28) suffered from chronic fatigue for twelve years. She was happily engaged but she felt a lack of motivation, and she was tired and depressed all the time. She avoided social contact because everything was too much effort for her. At least twice a week she had headaches with a stiff and sore neck, and pain in her shoulders and back. She needed long hours of sleep, but in the morning she did not feel refreshed. Some improvement could be felt from exercising but not for long periods. Her stomach was often bloated and she realized that it was worse from milk, bread, and wine. Her period was regular every month, but painful with cramps in the abdomen. In November 2002, an EAV test showed signals corresponding to Rickettsia coming from her immune system (Al), liver (F/LV), colon (GI/LI), spleen (RP/SP), and ovaries (V-8/UB-64). For balancing the meridians, the homeopathic remedy Veratrum album worked well.

Rx: Rickettsia mix 30 CH and Veratrum album 30 CH.

The diet for her excluded: sugar, fructose, dairy products, wheat, and alcohol (Table 4).

In January 2003 she felt better, and she realized that something had changed. She had more energy, better digestion, and she had headaches only from stress. The signal for Rickettsia came only from the spleen (RP/SP). We tested on this meridian to find a new balancing combination of remedies.

Rx: Rickettsia mix 30 CH, Chininum arsenicum 6 CH, and Cellfood drops, a source of oxygen.

She married in February and went on a happy honeymoon. Her digestion was good, but she still felt tired. In March the signal for Rickettsia was still in the meridian of the spleen (RP/SP). A new combination of remedies was found.

Rx: Arnica 30 CH and Rhus toxicodendron 30 CH, alternating every week.

The meridian of the spleen was cleared in May 2003, six months after the detection of Rickettsia. This case shows that the intracellular pathogens are difficult to clear. Waves and cycles of recovering from the infection can be expected, but there is no place for disappointment, as persistence will do the job.

Case 24 (862-2-187) (Eczema – protein indigestion)

Erika (32) had eczema continuously from the age of two years. It occurred worst of all on her palms. Lately the eczema had moved up the hands and as far as the elbows. This year she had had three periods of aggravation of her condition and each time she had felt weepy, with a lack of appetite, and dizzy and nauseous. She was very apprehensive of the fact that the eczema might start on her face, as dry, red spots above her upper lip had appeared. Her eczema was worse from contact with water. The girl was constipated. Her period was not regular. It used to come every two to three months. In February 1998 the EAV test revealed a very complicated picture. The liver (F/LV) and kidneys (R/KI) were normal. But the pancreas had very high readings at two points: (RP-1/SP-1, corresponding to proteolytic enzymes) and (RP-4/SP-2, corresponding to purine metabolism and uric acid diathesis). In addition, the meridian of the hormones (TR/TW) was in disorder, and so was the colon (GI/LI) and skin meridian (S/SK). A pathogen was not detected, but probably protein indigestion was the main cause of the eczema. A food test was done and it was suggested to the girl that she stop the intake of milk, cheese, butter, fish, red meat, chicken, peanuts, sunflower seeds, cashew nuts, coconuts, lentils, soy, and corn for three months. The best remedy for her eczema was Natrium muriaticum. In addition, hormonal nosodes were recommended.

Rx: Natrium muriaticum 30 CH, Ovarium 30 CH, and Thyreoidea 30 CH.

One month later she had a 70% improvement of the EAV reading and the eczema was very much reduced. A test of the affected meridians indicated that a new combination of natural remedies was required.

Rx: Sulphur 30 CH, Aristolochia/Ovaria comp, and Echinaforce drops.

Very soon her eczema disappeared and the hormones were normal. Three years later in 2001 she came in for a common diarrhea problem and she reported that since the treatment her eczema had never come back again.

Case 25 (5775-5-69) (Eczema – fungal infection)

Patty (28) suffered for one year with eczema on the palms of her hands. Three to four months previously it had spread to her arms and legs as big spots, very red on the edge and pink inside. In the center it started with little blisters, burning, itching, and peeling later. During the last month she had had patches on her face. She had a bloated abdomen, swollen legs, and a tendency toward depression. In June 2002 she was diagnosed by an EAV test with a mixed fungal infection. The signals appeared from her immune and lymphatic systems (Al, Ly), spleen (RP/SP), both kidneys (R/KI), and gallbladder (VB/GB). The liver was normal. An anti-fungal diet was suggested (Table 4).

Rx: Mixed nosode fungi 30 CH, Acidum phosphoricum 200 CH, and Sutherlandia (South African herbal immune-booster).

Three months later she was 60% better as judged by the reading of the meridians. The lady was strict about the diet as she felt that it worked, and her skin was much better.

Rx: Mixed nosode fungi 30 CH, Acidum nitricum 30 CH, and Sutherlandia.

In November 2002 her skin was clear. She was not strict with the diet anymore. She realized that drinking wine could cause the eczema to start again. The EAV reading of the meridians was normal.

Rx: Acidum nitricum 30 CH and the diet for one month more.

Seven months later in June 2003 she had very good readings for the meridians, no eczema, and no complaints.

Case 26 (4642-4-38) (Ulcerative colitis – fungi)

Isabelle (45) was diagnosed with ulcerative colitis in 1997 and suffered for five years. She constantly used the medications Lanzor and Asacol. She had acidity and heartburn from everything: food and drink, even from water. Often she had blood in her stools, bright red or brownish. She was tired and had headaches lately. At the beginning of May 2002 a colonoscopy showed a severe ulceration of the sigmoid part of her colon. On May 16, 2002, the EAV test detected a mixed fungal infection with signals coming from her immune system (Al), liver (F/LV), spleen (RP/SP), and colon (GI/LI). Her stomach (E/ST) and the small intestines (IG/SI) readings were normal. One remedy was enough to balance her meridians.

Rx: Aurum iodatum 6 CH. An anti-fungal diet was suggested (Table 4).

In August 2002 she was much better. The blood in her stools had disappeared. She still had heartburn, but she was delighted because the last colonoscopy (on June 20, 2002) showed a mild ulceration, not as severe as before. Objectively, the fungi still gave signals from the colon (GI/LI) and the spleen (RP/SP).

Rx: Aurum iodatum 6 CH.

On December 5, 2002, she was very well. She had no pain, and the stool was clear of blood. Then she reduced the conventional medicine. She was happy with the anti-fungal diet, because in seven months she had lost 10 kg and her weight had stabilized. Her organs were normal, and even the spleen and colon meridians were balanced. A treatment period of eight months had been necessary for clearing her system of fungi.

Case 27 (4591-4-30) (Fungi in the arteries)

Rudy (59) went through two coronary bypass operations in six months: in October 2001 and in April 2002. Cholesterol was not found, but sclerosis and blockage of the arteries was the problem. Heart problems were part of his family history and he had had hypertension for 15 years. In recent months he had often experienced flatulence. He used to take different allopathic medications constantly. His main concern was how to stop the process of sclerosis and blockage of his coronary arteries. On May 3, 2002, the Voll test detected a mixed fungal infection. The signals appeared from his immune and lymphatic systems (Al, Ly), liver (F/LV), spleen (RP/SP), and the point of the arteries (MC-1/CI-1). The presence of the fungi was confirmed by dark field microscopy examination of his blood. The Voll test indicated a combination of remedies that normalized the affected meridians.

Rx: Acidum fluoricum 6 CH and Nux vomica 30 CH.

An anti-fungal diet was suggested (Table 4). He was very strict with his diet and he took his homeopathic remedies regularly.

In July 2002 the EAV test showed that his system was clear of fungal infection. This was confirmed by dark field microscopy carried out on a live blood sample and by a general medical test with computer tomography.

Rx: Acidum fluoricum 6 CH and Barley green. It was suggested that he keep to the anti-fungal diet for as long as possible.

Case 28 (45 09-4-29) (A baby not growing well)

Marty (15 months) was born weighing 4.5 kg, but at the age of 15 months weighed only 9 kg. He was very often sick and on antibiotics. The child was very constipated, used to vomit a lot, had poor digestion, and was always in a bad mood. In April 2002 an EAV test was done. The measurements were made via the mother. (First the mother was tested, she was healthy, with normal readings for her meridians. After that the same measurements were done on her while she was holding the baby's hand.) The immune system of the child was good, and the lungs and the liver, too. Pathogens were not detected. Abnormal readings appeared from his lymphatic system (Ly) and his pancreas (points RP-1,3,5/SP-1,1b,3), which showed that the child had problems with the digestion of both carbohydrates and proteins. A food test was done and many foods appeared

198

to be difficult for him to digest: milk, cheese, yogurt, soy, red meat, pork meat, white bread, cake flower, corn, rice, sugar, fructose, honey, bananas, mango, and grapes. I suggested to his mother that these foods should be avoided for three months. One homeopathic remedy was enough to return the child's meridians to the normal condition.

Rx: Argentum nitricum 6 CH.

Three months later, in July 2002, the child showed a very great improvement in his digestive system. Now he had a good appetite, a bowel movement three times a day, and very good color in his face. He put on 1.5 kg of weight in three months regardless of the fact that he had had a respiratory infection during that time. Objectively, the meridian of the pancreas was normal. In December 2003 the parents informed me that the child had good digestion and was growing well. This is a very common kind of case, as lots of babies need support for their pancreas. The homeopathic remedy Argentum nitricum is good for the pancreatic function. I believe that after this treatment children will hardly ever develop intolerance to food or a food allergy.

Case 29 (3181-2-167) (Swollen extremities)

Taylor (60) had very swollen hands and feet for five months; they were red and sometimes even purple. The condition was worse in the mornings on waking, when it was difficult for him to hold anything, or even to walk. After some movement, it was better, but never back to normal. He went for blood tests, his heart was checked, and everything was normal. Generally, he was a healthy man, he had always had normal bowel movements and normal urination. He mentioned that he never used to drink water, but sweet soft drinks, at least two liters a day. In March 2001 he was tested by EAV. High signals appeared from his immune system (AI), lymphatic vessels (MC-9/CI-7b), liver (F/LV), spleen, and pancreas (RP/SP). A pathogen was not found. A food test showed that the main allergen for his system was sugar and everything sweet, including his soft drinks. After EAV testing, the following combination of natural remedies was recommended.

Rx: Argentum nitricum 30 CH, Water ease herbal tablets, and Potassium chloride to replace half of his salt intake.

One month later, in April 2001, he was 95% better. His hands and his feet were almost normal, as he explained "a little bit swollen only in the morning," but during the day he was very well. He was good at keeping to his "no sugar" diet. Objectively, his immune system, pancreas, and spleen were normal. Slightly high readings were detected from his lymphatic vessels point (MC/CI-9) and the liver (F/LV).

Rx: China 200 CH and Water ease tablets.

In June 2001 he had no more problems. I was sure that the EAV test had saved him from a serious sugar problem in the future.

Case 30 (2988-2-174) (Joint pain)

Will (73) suffered for 30 years from gout. During the latter six months it had been very bad. He had had severe pain in his left foot and in his right knee. The gentleman was very nervous and insisted on being helped about. He took allopathic medications for his gout and painkillers, but he needed something more. In November 2000 the EAV test revealed that his pancreas (RP/SP, right side) was his main problem. The other affected meridians were kidney (R/KI, left) and joints (Ad/JO). Pathogens were not found. A food test showed that he had to avoid some foods: red meat, nuts, milk, cheese, sugar, honey, watermelon, pineapple, bananas, oranges, tomatoes, spinach, kiwifruit, wine, tea, and whisky. After EAV testing, the following remedies were recommended.

Rx: Calcium phosphoricum 30 CH and Aurum metallicum 6 CH.

The medicine that balanced his meridians showed that he might have an imbalance of calcium in his body.

Six days later he came complaining about the diet: It made his life difficult. We did the test again, and his pancreas was so much better that he was persuaded to stay on the diet. In December and January he was well. In February for three days he had pain in his left knee. The test showed that his pancreas and his kidney were well. The remedies that worked for his joint meridian (Ad/JO) were the following typical remedies for rheumatic pain.

Rx: Thuja 30 CH, Calcium phosphoricum 30 CH, and Aurum metallicum 6 CH.

At the end of April 2001 he reported that he was in very good health, and that for the previous two months he had had no pain and no inflammation. An EAV test showed normal meridians. He insisted that the foods be tested again. The food test made him very happy: Only tomatoes, spinach, oranges, wine, and tea were foods that were not good for him. In September 2001 he informed me that for five months he had been very well, did not take allopathic medications, and had no complaints about his joints.

Case 31 (335-5-118) (Epstein–Barr Virus (EBV) with confused mind)

Daphne (61) was generally a healthy lady who used to come to me for her arthritis only twice a year. In December 2002 she visited me, because lately she felt that something was wrong. She was unstable and she had suddenly fallen down the stairs in her house and she did not have "a very clear brain." The EAV test found a signal for EBV from her spleen (RP/SP). She needed antiviral homeopathic medicine and support for her immune system.

Rx: Nosode EBV 30 CH, Cinnabaris 30 CH, and Immunoboost with Coenzyme Q-10.

One week later she announced that a blood test confirmed the presence of Epstein–Barr virus. She was cured in three months by repeating the combination of remedies. Six months later she was tested again, and according to the EAV test she was clear of the virus. Over the next two years I tested her spleen every three to four months, but it was perfectly clear.

Case 32 (6267-5-152) (EBV – miscarriages and memory problems)

Shana (33) had two children, she wanted another one, but she had had two miscarriages in two years. As a student in law school she had lots of exams but had difficulty concentrating. She was very tired and could not exercise lately. She had very hard, cracked heels, with deep cracks, which was strange because she never walked barefoot. In February 2003 by EAV test EBV was found affecting her liver and spleen. The hormones, the uterus, and the ovaries were normal. Her husband was tested. He had the same virus, affecting his spleen (RP/SP) and prostate gland (V-7/UB-65). A combination of remedies for Shana was found, but the last two of them clashed, so they could not be taken together.

Rx: EBV 30 CH, Mercurius bi-iodatus 6 CH, and Antimonium crudum 30 CH; the last two remedies to be alternated weekly.

For her husband who had the same virus, Mercurius vivus worked well.

Both of them were cured in three months. After three months, Shana explained that her memory had improved about four weeks after the beginning of the treatment. She wrote her exams in law successfully. Her energy was good, and she started running again, five kilometers three times a week.

Case 33 (5715-5-45) (EBV – depression and panic attacks)

Adeline (55) was diagnosed with EBV and she was given homeopathic medicine, but after nine months, in June 2002, she still felt the same symptoms: tired, agitated, hormonal imbalance, swollen ankles, nausea in the morning and during the day, depression, and panic attacks. EAV testing revealed that EBV was still present in her immune system (AI), spleen (RP/SP), liver (F/LI), kidneys (R/KI), and lymphatic vessels (MC-9/CI-7b). The best combination of remedies for balancing the meridians was the following.

Rx: EBV 30 CH, Antimonium crudum 200 CH, and South African herbal immune booster Sutherlandia.

After one month the homeopathic remedy Antimonium crudum 200 was replaced with Kalium arsenicosum 200 CH.

She was cured in four months. The signal for EBV and her symptoms vanished. After eight months she was tested again, and she had no complaints and no signal for EBV.

Case 34 (3600-5-5) (EBV – severe headaches)

Karina (34) had very severe headaches and vertigo, which were worse when bending down. First she was given an antidepressant, but it did not help. She was sleepy during the day and had nausea morning and evening. "Everything is as in a dream," she explained. In July 2001 by EAV test EBV was found.

The best medicine for this situation was Arsenicum album 200 CH and Cinnabaris 30 CH (to alternate every three days).

However, she was skeptical about homeopathic remedies and she did not take them. She was treated for more than a year for headache with conventional painkillers. In the end her doctor insisted that she be admitted to the hospital and she was treated there with antibiotics for ten days. But the headaches were unbearable.

After her hospital stay, she again came to see us. The signal for EBV was the same.

Rx: Mercurius solubilis 30 CH, six doses a day for a week, after that three doses a day.

This time she was good about taking her medicine.

She was cured in four months. The headaches stopped altogether, and the signal from EBV had vanished. Since then she has been well.

Case 35 (5857-5-61) (Coxsackie virus with headaches for many years)

Rodger (45) had headaches for eighteen years. He thought that it was because of a car accident he had had twenty years previously, and he used to go regularly for neck massage. It was helpful and eased the pain, but only for a short time. The headaches were of the migraine type: affecting half the head only, right or left, with disturbed vision during the attack. Very often the migraine appeared at night at about 1 a.m. and lasted through the next day. Rodger often had heartburn from wheat. He sometimes experienced pain in the area of the heart. Generally he did not complain of anything else; he felt healthy the rest of the time, when free of headaches. In July 2002 the EAV test showed five Coxsackie viruses of group B (types 2,3,4,5,6). The signals came from the immune and lymphatic systems (Al, Ly), pancreas (RP/SP right), spleen (RP/SP left), stomach (E/ST), and heart (C/HE). The recommended remedies included the following.

Rx: Coxsackie virus 30 CH, Mercurius solubilis 6 CH, Cactus grandiflorus 30 CH, and Carbo vegetabilis 30 CH.

An allergy test showed intolerance to many foods, including dairy products, sugar, bread, alcohol, chocolate, red meat, pork meat, eggs, and nuts, and he was asked to restrict those foods.

Two months later he reported that the headaches were gone and the heartburn was gone. He was strict with the diet, he lost 8 kg, and he was glad and proud of this. An EAV test showed normal signals from the lymphatic system, pancreas, spleen, and stomach. The signal for Coxsackie virus had disappeared. His food intolerance was reduced and he now had problems only with sugar, bread, and chocolate. The proteins were no longer a problem for his digestion.

After another two months he was still free of headaches, with a normal condition for everything but the heart. Signals from the heart points (C-7/HE-8a and C-8/HE-8) bothered me. He reported that he did sports, but I was concerned about the reading so I suggested a consultation with a cardiologist.

Case 36 (5876-5-88) (Coxsackie virus with chest pain)

Saundra (15) had Coxsackie virus as diagnosed by a blood test 15 months previously. The results showed group B viruses. She was on painkillers for a persistent sharp pain in the upper chest. During the day she had hot flushes, headaches, dizziness, and nausea. Lately she felt pain around the heart. Her menses had not been regular for a year. She felt constantly tired. In July 2002 an EAV test confirmed Coxsackie group B viruses (B-1,2,5,6). The signals came from the lymphatic system (Ly), spleen (RP/SP), stomach (E/ST), kidneys (R/KI), right ovary (V-8/UB-64), hormones (TR/TW), nerves (Nd/NE), and heart (C/HE). She was cured in three months with the following combination.

Rx: Coxsackie 200 CH, Mercurius vivus 30 CH, Vitamin C, and a complex of vitamins and minerals named Immunoguard.

She was free of headaches, pain in the chest, with a normal period and normal EAV readings for everything tested. Two months later she had nausea after every meal. The test for Coxsackie virus was negative. She had a signal for Helicobacter pylori and she was given Arsenicum album 30 CH with good results.

Case 37 (4286-4-56) (Coxsackie virus with Lymphoedema)

Lilia (47) was very sick with swollen legs, and a big, puffy body. When she came in during February 2002, she really looked unwell: puffy, pale, tired, exhausted, and weepy. Two years previously she was diagnosed with Lymhpoedema, but the cause was unknown. In two years she had put on 18 kilograms of weight, the roots of her hair were inflamed, and she had headaches at least once a week. Her mother was very concerned about her health, and she showed me 12 different medications that she was taking at that time, which did not improve her condition. The EAV test showed that the liver, gallbladder, and kidneys were normal. Coxsackie viruses were found, expressed by the reading from the immune and lymphatic systems (Al, Ly), high signals from the spleen (RP/SP), and a very high reading at the point MC-9/CI-7b for lymphatic vessels. The medicines for balancing her system were the following.

Rx: Coxsackie vir. mixed nosode 30 CH and Mercurius vivus 6 CH in combination with Vitamin C.

One month later she felt much better, not so swollen anymore. The reading for the other organs was better, but not for the kidneys. An infection with the bacteria E-coli was found.

Rx: Mercurius vivus 6 CH, E-coli 30 CH, and Cantarris 30 CH.

After a food test, it was found that many foods such as cheese, sugar, fructose, bread, pasta, rice, maize, oats, Coca-Cola, bananas, grapes, tea, and alcohol had to be avoided.

In the following two months, she improved dramatically. The signal from the virus diminished in July 2002, five months after the beginning of the treatment. Everything tested was normal, she felt very well. She lost weight and she looked very good. Three months later in October 2002 she was tested again and everything was normal. The food test showed that she had to keep to a "no sugar" diet.

Case 38 (6245-5-156) (Coxsackie virus with muscle spasms of the throat)

Roslyn (52) could not swallow liquids. On August 5, 2002, she took a sip of water and felt painful spasms, and since then for the past six months she could not swallow any liquids normally, only very small sips could pass down her throat, but not one after another. She could hardly drink a glass of water a day and she was in despair. She was on tranquilizers. And she felt so tired and exhausted those six months that she could not do her work efficiently. She used to do charity work, helping very ill people: cancer, AIDS, and TB patients. But now she was very weak, thin, and losing weight, and she only wanted to sleep. The EAV test revealed a very irritated immune and lymphatic system (Al, Ly) and spleen (RP). Many types of Coxsackie virus were present: B1 to B6, A2 and A7. The following combination of natural remedies was recommended.

205

Rx: Mercurius corrosivus 30 CH, Coxsackie vir 30 CH, and Food form antioxidant.

Two months later she was still tired and she could not swallow properly. Generally she was much more relaxed, she had put on 2 kg, and she looked better. Objectively, her EAV reading had improved by 30%. It was interesting to me that at that time signals from her immune, lymphatic system, and spleen (Al, Ly, RP/SP) reacted positively to the homeopathic nosode Syphillinum. Probably a new energy layer had opened a syphilitic miasmatic influence in her system.

Rx: Syphillinum 200 CH, Phosphorus 30 CH, Mercurius solubilis 30 CH, and homeopathic Antiviral mix (with homeopathic Interferon and γ-Globulin), and Antioxidant.

In June 2003, four months after the first visit, she could swallow well: She could drink 500 ml in five minutes. She was not as tired as before, and not sleepy anymore. She had a nice rosy color on her face. She said: "I have sparkles in my eyes now," and she was very thankful.

Rx: Mercurius iodatus flavus 200 CH, Mercurius solubilis 30 CH, and Syphillinum 200 CH for another month.

After a further two months she was so well that she decided to travel to Tibet.

Case 39 (4436-5-103) (Cytomegalo virus (CMV) with hormonal imbalance)

Elda (35) was not well for 14 months. During that period she was diagnosed with hypothyroidism and ovarian cysts. The problem had started with a sore throat for two months and flu-like symptoms. During the last year her menstruation had occurred once in three months. She was on medication for the thyroid gland (Eltroxin 0.05 mg). She was putting on weight, and was pale, tired, exhausted, and unhappy. In March 2002 by EAV test CMV was found with signals from her immune system (Al), thyroid and pituitary glands (TR-7/TW-2, TR-8/TW-3, right side), liver (F/LV), spleen (RP/SP), and both her ovaries (V-8/UB-64).

Rx: CMV 30 CH, Mercurius vivus 30 CH, Modu Care (an immuno-modulator), and Vitamin C.

One month later menstruation came on time. Objectively, the hormones and the ovaries were normal. The immune system and the spleen were much better. A signal from the colon appeared, responding to the tester for Enterococcus bacteria. The liver gave signals for toxins.

Rx: Arsenicum album 30 CH, Mercurius vivus 30 CH, Mercurius solubilis 30 CH, CMV 30 CH, Modu Care, and Vitamin C.

In June 2002, after three months of homeopathic treatment she felt well, with more energy. Her menstruation was very frequent, every two weeks. Objectively, she still had CMV (signals from the spleen), Enterococcus in the colon, an irritated liver, and weakness of the thyroid gland. She needed a very complex medicine to adequately rebalance the meridians.

Rx: Arsenicum iodatum 30 CH, CMV 30 CH, Mercurius solubilis 30 CH, Causticum 30 CH, Modu Care, and Vitamin C.

In September 2002, five months after the beginning of her treatment, her condition was good, free of CMV, with normal signals for every organ of her body. During the following ten months she was tested periodically and she was well.

Case 40 (4393-4-44) (Cytomegalo virus (CMV) with imbalance of the pancreas)

Lacy (39) was tired for eight months, sleepy during the day, and exhausted in the evening. She had become sensitive to organic chemicals. She went to her doctor and lots of tests were done. The blood test showed a high level of insulin for unknown reasons. Vitamin B injections were prescribed but with no result, and her condition stayed the same. In March 2002 the EAV test showed CMV with signals from her immune system (AI), spleen (RP/SP left), right kidney (R/KI), and the pancreas (irritated points in the right side RP-3,5/SP-1b,3), related to sugar digestion. The food test showed intolerance to: sugar, fructose, sweet fruits, chicken, beer, and tobacco.

Rx: CMV 30 CH, Mercurius solubilis 30 CH, and Vitamin C 1,000 mg.

In two months she was cleared of CMV and the food intolerances disappeared in three months. During the next five months she was tested periodically, but there were no signals for the presence of the virus.

Case 41 (4584-4-46) (CMV with protein indigestion)

Jasper (40) was a marathon runner, but recently had been waking up in the morning with headaches, fatigue, and with a sore lower back. This condition persisted and worsened over more than three months. Before this he had felt strong and was used to running long distances every morning. Lately he could not do his training exercises, and he was afraid that he would not be able to take part in the marathon competitions that year. In April 2002 an EAV test found CMV. The signals appeared from his lymphatic system (Ly), liver (F/LV), spleen (RP-1/SP-1, left side), pancreas (the point RP-1/SP-1 right side), and the thyroid gland, right side (TR-7/TW-2). The food test showed that red meat, peanuts, vinegar, wine, spirits, coffee, and Coca-Cola must be avoided. The recommendation was as follows.

Rx: CMV 30 CH, Mercurius corrosivus 12 CH, in combination with Vitamin C.

In June 2002, after two months, the headaches stopped. His lymphatic system, liver, pancreas, and thyroid gland became normal. The virus was still there, giving signals from the spleen. The food test showed that red meat and peanuts were not a problem any longer. The homeopathic medicine was continued for a further two months, and after that, in September 2002, the virus disappeared. A week later he reported that he was in very good health and that he had run a distance of 50 km. After four months, in January 2003, he was tested again and everything was in perfect condition.

Case 42 (6115/6133-5-185) (A young couple with infertility)

Freida (28) came to me in November 2002 with an infertility problem she had had for two years. She had been put on hormonal treatments, but still had no result. Generally she was sleepy, tired, and with irregular menstruation. The EAV test showed that her hormonal system gave normal signals. Strong signals for CMV appeared from her immune system (Al), lymphatic system (Ly), spleen (RP/SP), and both kidneys (R/KI).

Rx: CMV 30 CH, Cinnabaris 200 CH, and Stimulandia (a herbal immune booster).

I suggested that her husband should also be tested.

Her husband (29) was tested by blood tests for hormones and the results revealed a low level of testosterone, which was connected with a disturbed function of the pituitary gland. At that time a blood test revealed high cholesterol. He was tired and of late restless. He had difficulty falling asleep and he used to wake up two or three times during the night. For two years he had had itchy skin all over his body, and during the latter year he had put on 5 kg of weight. The EAV test showed a very complicated picture. He had signals for CMV from his spleen (RP/SP-left) and right testicle (V-8/UB-64), but the immune system (Al), liver, pancreas (F/LV, RP/SP-right), pituitary gland (TR-8/TW-3), and the spleen (RP/SP-left) gave signals for mixed viral infections of Coxsackie and Epstein–Barr viruses. The pancreas had strong signals for sugar and protein indigestion (RP-1,5/SP-1,3), and the liver was seriously affected (F-1 to 5/LV-1 to 2a).

Rx: Mixed antiviral nosode for three viruses (CMV, Coxsackie virus, EBV) 30 CH, Mercurius iodatus flavus 6 CH, and Coenzyme Q-10.

I suggested that they should not try to conceive during the treatment for the viruses.

The family came for a followup visit two months later. Freida still had a signal for CMV in her spleen, but the other organs were normal: immune system, lymphatic system, and kidneys.

Rx: Mixed antiviral nosode 30 CH (CMV, Coxsackie virus, EBV) and Mercurius cyanatus 30 CH.

Freida's husband continued to have signals for viruses in his spleen, but everything else was normal: immune system, left testicle, liver, and pancreas.

Rx: Mixed antiviral nosode 30 CH and Mercurius solubilis 30 CH.

At the end of February 2003, four months after the beginning of their treatment, they both were clear of viruses. I repeated their remedies for one more month. In the beginning of July they telephoned me to say that Freida was ten weeks pregnant and that she was very well. At the beginning of December she was seven months pregnant and very well and happy. Two months later she gave birth to a healthy baby girl. The family visited me with the baby, and I still keep a photograph of the beautiful baby in a pink dress.

Case 43 (4320-3-48) (Rotavirus with lymphatic stasis)

Madeleine (45) had had pain and pressure in the area of her spleen for at least two years. She experienced heaviness and water retention with swollen legs, and she had lumps under the skin of the upper legs. She felt "as if the lymph did not move." For a long time she was tired, even in the morning. In addition she had osteoporosis with pain in the left hip. She

209

had been taking a calcium preparation and hormone replacement therapy, but still she did not feel well. She had a bowel movement two to three times a day, always very soft. In February 2002 she was tested by EAV. Signals for Rotavirus were found coming from her immune and lymphatic system (AI, Ly), spleen (RP/SP), gallbladder (VB/GB), left lung (P/LU), and the lymph vessels (MC-9/CI-7b). The meridian of the joints (Ad/JO) had a high reading, reacting positively to the homeopathic remedy Calcarea carbonica.

Rx: Rotavirus 30 CH, Carbo vegetabilis 30 CH, and Calcarea carbonica 200 CH.

Two months later she reported that she felt there was great improvement: The pressure in the spleen was no longer there and she explained "The lymph is moving now." Objectively, she had no signal for the virus anymore from her immune system, spleen, gallbladder, and left lung. The reading in the point of the lymph vessels (MC-9/CI-7b) was still high. The joint meridian was normal. She wanted me to test her hormones, because she felt moody and had a low sex drive. The EAV test found slightly high readings for the thyroid gland, both sides (TR-7/TW-2).

Rx: Thyreoidea 30 CH, Estrogen 200 CH, and Carbo vegetabilis 30 CH.

In June 2002, four months after the first visit, the lumps under the skin of her legs had disappeared, but she felt pressure in the spleen again. She felt very well after taking the medicine for her hormones (homeopathic Thyreoidea and Estrogen), and now she was in a better mood and her sex drive increased. The EAV measurements showed normal readings for the immune and lymphatic systems, the hormones were normal, but again one signal for Rotavirus from her spleen was found, at point RP-1/SP-1.

Rx: Rotavirus 30 CH and Mercurius solubilis 200 CH.

After that the meridian of the spleen was balanced and she had no more complaints.

Case 44 (A child without hair)

Michael was six years old, but he had never had hair, eyebrows, or eyelashes. His mother was my client, and she just mentioned him and asked if something could be done. She explained that she was a single mother, Michael was her second child, and she had not wanted him.

During the pregnancy, she even tried to abort him with drugs, but the child survived. I asked her to bring Michael with her the next time she came for her consultation. He was a shy child and looked at me as if he was begging me to excuse him from occupying my attention. I tested him with EAV. Michael's organs were all absolutely healthy, only a signal from the emotional point on the meridian of the heart (MC-1/HE-9, left side) was high. The signal was balanced with the homeopathic remedy Stramonium 200 CH, a remedy given for extreme stress with fear, horror, and violence. This remedy is given to a person who feels that his life is in danger. Perhaps the child had known and had understood what was happening while he was in his mother's womb.

Rx: Stramonium 200 CH, one dose in the evening, once a week for one to two months.

During the next consultation a month later the mother reported that she had given him the remedy as recommended. She also mentioned that the child became gentle with her, and he started giving her hugs and kisses. I did not know before that the child did not want to kiss her. After six months the mother came to thank me. She was happy that Michael's hair had started growing. I keep a photograph of little Michael with his blond hair.

APPENDICES

TABLE 3
BACTERIAL AND FUNGAL PATHOGENS AND HOMEOPATHIC REMEDIES CONFIRMED BY EAV TESTS AS SPECIFIC FOR THESE PATHOGENS

PATHOGEN	HOMEOPATHIC REMEDY
Aerobacter	Ac-pic., Arg-n., Ars., Bry.
Aspergillus	Ac-citr., Ac-carb., Ac-fl., Ac-n., Ac-p., Ac-pic., Ac-sul., Aur-met., Aur-i., Aur-mur., Bism-met., Bism-subn., Caust., Phos. (and oxidants)
Bacillus coli	Podo.*, Aur-mur., Aur-sul.
Bacillus dysenterium	Bapt.*, Aur-mur.
Bacillus Morgan	Lach.
Borrellia	Ars-iod.
Bordetella pertussis	Ant-t, Drosera
Brucella melitensis	Card-mar*, Colch., Caust.
Campylobacter & Helicobacter	Anac.*, Alum., Ars., Ars-iod., Bism-met., Bism-subn., Cadm-met., Chelid., Hyper., Phos., Zn-met., Zn-phos., Verat. (and oxidants)
Candida	Ac-pic., Ac-carbol., Ac-lact., Ac-fl., Aur-iod, Bellis-per., Borax, Phos., Pyrog. (Vit. C and antioxidants)
Chlamidia	Con., Rumex*, Ac-n., Acon., Ac-sul-fl., Aeth., Ac-pic., Agar., Arg-nit., Bry., Kali-i., Kreos., Lach., Merc-v., Merc-cy., Pyrog., Sabina, Sanic. (Vit. B, Vit. C, and antioxidants)
Clostridium diffic.	Ac-carbol., Ac-n., Ac-p., Ac-sarcol., Ac-fl., Ac-pic., Ac-sul., Arg-n., Ars-i., Ars-sul-fl., Borax, Bism-met., Cupr-met., Gels., Hep., Kali-bi., Kali-i., Merc-corr., Nux-v. (and oxidants)

213

Table 3 (continued)

PATHOGEN	HOMEOPATHIC REMEDY
Cryptococcus	Anac.*, Ac-carbol., Ac-p., Ars., Aur-i., Bism-met., Bism-subn., Bry., Kali-i., Merc-sol. (and oxidants)
E-coli	Ac-benz., Ac-pic., Arundo, Canth., Chrom-kali-sulph., Chin-ars., Kali-br., Kali-i., Mercury salts (and oxidants; Colloidal silver)
Enterobacteria	Kali-ars., Kali-bi., Kali-s. (and oxidants)
Enterococcus	Ars., Ars-i., Bry., Chin-ars., Hydrastis*, Lyc., Nat-ars., Phos., Sarsap. (and oxidants)
Gardnerella	Canth., Clematis, Equis., Merc-sol., Sarsap. (and Vit. B)
Helicobacter	(see Campylobacter)
Haemoph. infl.	Ars., Chelid. (and oxidants)
Klebsiella	Ant-t., Ars., Lobelia, Sticta. (Vit. C and antioxidants)
Listeria monocyt.	Merc-corr.
Meningococcus	Adonis-v.*, Hyosc.*, Mercury salts
Mucor	Ac-benz., Ac-citr., Ac-carbol., Ac-fl., Ac-n., Ac-p., Ac-pic., Ac-sarcol., Ac-sul., Ars., Ars-i., Aur-met., Aur-i., Aur-mur., Bism-met., Bism-subn., Caust., Phos. (and oxidants)
Mycoplasma & Ureaplasma	Equisetum*, Ars., Ars-i., Chlor., Graph., Kali-ars., Kali-br., Kali-c., Kali-i., Kali-p., Phos., Pyrog., Spong., Sticta. (Vit. B, Vit. C, and antioxidants)
Mycobacterium tuberculosis	Laur., Kreos.*, Scroful.*, Mercury salts, Phos., Tub. (and oxidants)
Pneumococcus	Kali-bi.*, Kali-sul.*, Kali-ars., Kali-c., Kali-mur., Nat-ars., (see also Streptococcus)
Propionbacterium acne	Lach.

Table 3 (continued)

PATHOGEN	HOMEOPATHIC REMEDY
Proteus	Cinnab.*, Ac-n., Aur-i., Aur-met., Aur-mur., Clem., Mez., Phos., Pyrog., Sep.
Pseudomonas	Bry., China. (and oxidants)
Rickettsia	Ac-mur., Arn., Agar., Apis, Ars., Ars-i., Aur-sul., Bapt., Bellis-p., Bry., Carb-v., Chel., Chin., Chin-ars., Colch., Crot-hor., Ign., Lach., Merc-cy., Verat. (Vit. B. and oxidants)
Salmonella	Verat.*, Ars., Ars-i. (and oxidants)
Serratia	Tereb., Thuja.
Shigella	Carb-v., Chin-ars., Cupr-ac., Cupr-met. (and antioxidants)
Staphylococcus	Cactus*, Conv.*, Phyt.*, Sil.*, Stroph.*, Ant-ars., Chin-ars., Coff., Hep., Kali-bi., Mercury salts (and oxidants)
Streptococcus	Crat.*, Diosc.*, Phyt.*, Urt-u.*, Ac-sul., Ars., Bellis-p., Kali-ars., Merc-cy., Merc-sol., Merc-v., Phos., Rhus-t., Sticta., Puls. (see also Pneumococcus)
Streptomyces	Ac-fl.
Termibacterium	Hydrastis, Kali-mur.
Trichophytie	Ac-n., Ac-carbol., Ac-fl., Ac-mur., Aur-met., Aur-i., Bism-met., Bism-subn. (and oxidants)
Ureaplasma	(see Mycoplasma)
Yersinia	Kreos.*, Ars-i., Bism-met., Bism-subn., Bufo, Calc-i., Chin., Cinnab., Hep., Hydrastis, Kali-bi., Mag-mur., Thuja, Verat. (and oxidants)

According to Usupov, G. A. (2000)

TABLE 4
BACTERIAL AND FUNGAL PATHOGENS
RELATED TO FOOD INTOLERANCE

A-Alcohol, **D**-Dairy products, **F**-Fructose, **S**-Sugar, **V**-vinegar, **W**-Wheat.

PATHOGEN	INTOLERANCE	EXCEPTIONS
Aerobacter coli	A+D+F+S+V	
Aspergillus	A+D+F+S+V+W Soy+Vit B+Starch	Butter+Rice+Yogurt
Bacillus coli	A+F+S+V	
Bacillus dysent.	A+D+S+V	
Borrellia	A+D+S+V	Butter+Yogurt
Campylobacter & Helicobacter	A+D+S+V+Soy	Butter+Yogurt
Candida (antifungal diet)	A+D+F+S+V+W Soy+Vit B+ Starch	Butter+Rice+Yogurt
Clostridium	A+D+S+V+W+Soy	F+Rye+Yogurt
Chlamidia	A+V+W	
Cryptococcus	A+D+F+S+V+W Soy+Vit B+Starch	Butter+Rice+Yogurt
E-coli	A+S+V	
Enterococcus	A+D+S+V	Yogurt
Gardnerella	A+S+V+W	
Gonococcus	A+S+V	
Klebsiella	A+D+F+S+V	
Mucor	A+D+F+S+V+W Soy+Vit B+Starch	Butter+Rice+Yogurt
Mycobact. tub.	A+S+V	
Mycoplasma	A+F+S+V+Soy	

Table 4 (continued)

PATHOGEN	INTOLERANCE	EXCEPTIONS
Propionbact. acne	A+F+S+V+W+Rye	
Proteus	A+D+S+V	Butter+Yogurt
Pseudomonas	A+D+S+V	
Rickettsia	A+D+S+V+W+Soy	F+Rye+Yogurt
Salmonella	A+D+S+V+W+Starch	Yogurt
Serratia	A+F+S+V+Soy	
Shigella	A+D+F+S+V	Yogurt
Staphylococcus	A+D+F+S+V	Yogurt
Streptococcus	A+D+F+S+V	Yogurt
Streptomyces	A+S+V	
Termibacter	A+D+F+S+V+W	
Ureaplasma	A+F+S+V+Soy	
Yersinia	A+D+F+S+V	

TABLE 5
SOME VIRUSES AND HOMEOPATHIC REMEDIES
SPECIFIC FOR THEM AS PROVED BY EAV TESTS

VIRUSES	HOMEOPATHIC REMEDIES
Adenoviruses	Bar-c.*
Coxsackie	Arn., Aur-sul., Hydrastis, Mercury salts: Cinnab., Merc-corr., Merc-cy., Merc-dul., Merc-i-fl., Merc-i-rub., Merc-sol., Merc-v.
Cytomegalo	Caust.*, Rhus-t.*, Arg-met., Ferr-i., Teucr., Mercury salts: Cinnab., Merc-corr., Merc-cy., Merc-dul., Merc-i-fl., Merc-i-rub., Merc-sol., Merc-v.
Epstein-Barr	Ant-c., Ars-i., Gels., Glon., Kali-ars., Nat-ars., Mercury salts: Cinnab., Merc-corr., Merc-cy., Merc-dul., Merc-i-fl., Merc-i-rub., Merc-sol., Merc-v.
Grippe	Cuprum-met., Mercury salts: Cinnab., Merc-corr., Merc-cy., Merc-dul., Merc-i-fl., Merc-i-rub., Merc-sol., Merc-v.
Herpes*	Ac-mur., Ars., Bufo., Caust., Clem., Croton-t., Digit., Dulc., Hep., Kreos., Nat-mur., Petr., Psor., Rhus-t., Sep., Stroph., Sulph., Tell., Thuja
Hepatitis	Card-mar*, Carb-an., Cab-v., Carb-s., Chel., Chin., Chin-ars., Chin-sul., Colch., Hydrastis, Merc-corr., Merc-sol., Nux-v.
Human Papillomavirus (HPV)	Mercury salts, Teucr., Visc-alb.
Polio	Lathyrus, Mercury salts: Cinnab., Merc-corr., Merc-cy., Merc-dul., Merc-i-fl., Merc-i-rub., Merc-sol., Merc-v.
Rotaviruses	Carb-v., Podo, Mercury salts: Cinnab., Merc-corr., Merc-cy., Merc-dul., Merc-i-fl., Merc-i-rub., Merc-sol., Merc-v.

According to Usupov, G. A. (2000)

TABLE 6
HOMEOPATHIC REMEDIES ACTIVE FOR DIFFERENT
PATHOGENS AND THEIR RESONANCE FREQUENCIES

HOMEOPATHIC REMEDY	PATHOGEN	RESONANCE FREQUENCIES KHz†
Ac-acet.	Amoebae	438, 385-398 (438-398)
Ac-benz.	Mucor	288, 353-392*
Ac-carbol.	Aspergillus Clostridium diff. Cryptococcus Mucor Trichophytie	325-385* 362-396 353-420 288, 353-392 184-325 (184-420)
Ac-citr.	Aspergillus Mucor	325-385 288, 353-392 (288-392)
Ac-fl.	Aspergillus Clostridium Mucor Streptomyces Trychophytie	325-385* 362-396 288, 353-392* n.a. 184-325* (128-325)
Ac-lact.	Candida	386
Ac-mur.	Rickettsia Herpes vir. Trichophytie	128-361* 291-325 184-325* (128-325)
Ac-nit.	Aspergillus Chlamidia Clostridium Mucor Proteus Trichophytie	325-385* 379-384 362-396 288; 353-392* 324-413 184-325* (184-413)

Table 6 (continued)

HOMEOPATHIC REMEDY	PATHOGEN	RESONANCE FREQUENCIES KHz†
Ac-phos.	Amoebae Aspergillus Clostridium diff. Cryptococcus Mucor	438, 385-398 325-385* 362-396 353-420* 288; 353-392* (288-420)
Ac-pic.	Aerobacter Aspergillus Candida Chlamidia Clostridium E-coli Mucor	374 325-385* 366 379-384 362-396 356-392 288; 353-392* (288-420)
Ac-sarc.	Clostridium Mucor	362-396 288; 353-392* (288-396)
Ac-sulph.	Aspergillus Clostridium Mucor	325-385* 362-396 288; 353-392 (288-392)
Ac-sul-fl.	Chlamydia	379-384
Adonis-vern.	Meningococcus	n.a.
Aconitum	Chlamydia	379-384
Aethusa	Chlamydia	379-384
Agaricus	Chlamydia	379-384
Aloe	Amoebae	438; 385-398

Table 6 (continued)

HOMEOPATHIC REMEDY	PATHOGEN	RESONANCE FREQUENCIES KHz†
Alumina	Campylobacter & Helicobacter	355-381
Anac.	Campylobacter & Helicobacter Cryptococcus	355-381 353-420* (353-420)
Ant-ars.	Staphylococcus	376-381
Ant-crud.	EBV	380
Ant-t.	Klebsiella Schistosoma (Bilharzia) Rickettsia Echinococcus	416-422 353-473 128-361* n. a.
Apis	Rickettsia Echinococcus	128-136* n.a.
Arg-met.	CMV	408-411
Arg-n.	Aerobacter Chlamydia Clostridium diff.	374 379-384 362-396 (362-396)
Ars-alb.	Aerobacter/ Enterobacter Cryptococcus Campylobacter/Helicobacter Enterococcus Herpes vir. Klebsiella Mucor Rickettsiae Salmonella Streptococcus	374 353-420* 355-368 325* 291-420 401-417 288, 353-392* 128-361* 329-355 318-385 (128-420)

Table 6 (continued)

HOMEOPATHIC REMEDY	PATHOGEN	RESONANCE FREQUENCIES KHz†
Ars-iod.	Borrellia	378-382
	Campylobacter	355-368
	Clostridium diff.	362-396
	Cryptococcus	353-421*
	Enterococcus	325*
	EBV	372-383
	Helicobacter	355-368
	Mucor	288, 353-392*
	Mycoplasma	323-343
	Rickettsiae	128-361*
	Yersinia	184-378*
		(184-396)
Ars-s-fl.	Clostridium diff.	362-396
	Chlamydia	379-384
		(362-396)
Aur-iod.	Aspergillus	325-385*
	Candida	385
	Cryptococcus	353-420*
	Mucor	288; 353-392*
	Proteus	324-413
	Trichophytie	184-325*
		(184-420)
Aur-met.	Aspergillus	325-385*
	Proteus	324-413
	Mucor	288; 353-392*
	Trichophytie	184-325*
		(184-413)

Table 6 (continued)

HOMEOPATHIC REMEDY	PATHOGEN	RESONANCE FREQUENCIES KHz†
Aur-mur.	Aspergillus	325-385*
	Bac. Coli	n.a.
	Bac. dysent.	n.a.
	Mucor	288; 353-392*
	Proteus	324-413
		(288-413)
Aur-sulph.	Coxsackie vir.	360-366
	Bac. Coli	n.a.
	Rickettsia	128-361*
		(360-366)
Bar-c.	Adenoviruses	n.a.
Baptisia	Bac. dysent.	n.a.
	Rickettsia	128-361*
Bellis-per.	Streptococcus	318-385
	Rickettsia	128-361*
		(128-385)
Berberis	Guiardia lamblia	421-426
Bism-met.	Aspergillus	325-385*
	Campylobacter	355-368
	Clostridium diff.	362-396
	Cryptococcus	353-420*
	Helicobacter	355-368
	Mucor	288; 353-392*
	Pseudomonas aer.	333
	Trichophytie	184-325*
	Yersinia	184-378*
		(184-420)

Table 6 (continued)

HOMEOPATHIC REMEDY	PATHOGEN	RESONANCE FREQUENCIES KHz†
Bism-subn.	Aspergillus	325-385*
	Campylobacter	355-368
	Cryptococcus	353-420*
	Helicobacter	355-368
	Mucor	288; 353-392*
	Trichophytie	184-325*
	Yersinia	184-378*
		(184-420)
Borax	Candida	386
	Clostridium diff.	362-396
	Malaria	372-442
		(372-442)
Bryonia	Aerobacter	374
	Amoebae	438; 385-398
	Chlamydia	379-384
	Clostridium diff.	362-396
	Cryptococcus	353-420*
	Pseudomonas aer.	406*; 331-335
	Rickettsia	128-361*
	Yersinia	184-378*
		(128-420)
Bufo	Herpes	291-420
	Yersinia	184-378
		(184-420)
Cadm-met.	Campylobacter	355-368
	Helicobacter	355-368
Calc-c.	Enterobius	423
Calc-iod.	Yersinia	184-378*
Cantaris	E-coli	365-392

224

Table 6 (continued)

HOMEOPATHIC REMEDY	PATHOGEN	RESONANCE FREQUENCIES KHz†
Carb-an.	Hepatitis	418
Carb-v.	Amoebae Hepatitis B Malaria Rotavirus Rickettsia Shigella	438; 385-391 418 372-442 n.a. 128-361* 318-398 (128-442)
Carb-s.	Hepatitis vir.	414-421
Card-mar.	Brucella mel. Hepatitis	n.a. 414-421
Caust.	Aspergillus Brucella mell. Herpes vir. Mucor	325-385* n.a. 291-420 288; 353-392* (128-420)
Cean-amer.	Clostridium diff.	362-396
Chelidonium	Clostridium diff. Hepatitis vir.	362-396 414-421 (362-421)
China	Babesia Clostridium diff. Hepatitis vir. Malaria Pseudomonas Rickettsia Yersinia	n.a. 362-396 414-421 372-442 406* 331-335 128-361* 184-378* (184-442)

Table 6 (continued)

HOMEOPATHIC REMEDY	PATHOGEN	RESONANCE FREQUENCIES KHz†
Chin-ars.	Hepatitis vir.	414-421
	Malaria	372-442
	EBV	376-383
	Enterococcus	325*
	E-coli	356-392
	Rickettsia	128-361*
	Shigella	356-392
	Staphylococcus	376-381
		(128-442)
Chin-sulph.	Hepatitis vir.	414-421
	Malaria	372-442
		(372-442)
China	Ascaris	403-410
	Enterobius	420-427
	Toxoplasma	395
		(395-427)
Chlorinum	Mycoplasma	423-434
Cinnabaris	EBV	376-383
	E-coli	356-392
	CMV	409
	Coxsackie vir.	360-366
	Meningococcus	n.a.
	Mycobact tub.	430-434
	Proteus	324-413
	Rotavirus	n.a.
	Staphylococcus	376-381
	Yersinia	184-378*
		(184-409)

Table 6 (continued)

HOMEOPATHIC REMEDY	PATHOGEN	RESONANCE FREQUENCIES KHz†
Clematis	Gardnerella Herpes vir. Proteus Trichomonas	338-343 291-420 324-413 378-384 (291-420)
Coffea	Staphylococcus	376-381
Colch.	Brucella Hepatitis Rickettsia	n.a. 414-421 128-361* (128-421)
Conium	Chlamydia	379-384
Crataegus	Streptococcus	318-385
Crot-hor.	Rickettsia	128-361*
Crot-tigr.	Herpes vir.	291-420
Cuprum-ars.	Shigella	310-394
Cuprum-met.	Clostridium diff. Grippe vir. Shigella Babesia	362-396 313-324 310-394 n.a. (310-396)
Digitalis	Herpes vir.	291-420
Dioscorea	Streptococcus	318-385
Dulcamara	Herpes vir. Mycoplasma & Ureaplasma	291-420 323-343 (291-420)

Table 6 (continued)

HOMEOPATHIC REMEDY	PATHOGEN	RESONANCE FREQUENCIES KHz†
Equisetum	Gardnerella Mycoplasma & Ureaplasma	338-343 323-343 (323-343)
Ferr-iod.	CMV	409
Gelsemium	Clostridium diff. EBV	362-396 376-383 (362-386)
Glonoinum	EBV	376-383
Graphytes	Mycoplasma & Ureaplasma	323-343
Helonias	Trichmonas hom.	378-384
Hepar-s.	Clostridium diff. Herpes vir. Staphylococcus Yersinia	362-396 291-420 376-381 184-378* (184-420)
Hydrastis	Coxsackie vir. Echinococcus Enterococcus Hepatitis vir. Termibacter Yersinia	360-366 441-462 325* 414-421 n.a. 184-378* (184-462)
Hyosciamus	Meningococcus	n.a.
Hypericum	Campylobacter & Helicobacter	355-368
Ignatia	Rickettsia	128-361*

Table 6 (continued)

HOMEOPATHIC REMEDY	PATHOGEN	RESONANCE FREQUENCIES KHz†
Kali-ars.	Hepatitis	414-421
	EBV	372-383
	Enterbacter/Aerobacter	374
	Enterococcus	325*
	Mycoplasma & Ureaplasma	324-343
	Pneumococcus	318-385
		(372-421)
Kali-bi.	Clostridium diff.	362-396
	Enterobacter/Aerobacter	374
	Pneumococcus	318-385
	Staphylococcus	376-381
	Yersinia	184-378*
		(184-396)
Kali-br.	E-coli	356-392
	Mycoplasma & Ureaplasma	323-343
		(323-392)
Kali-c.	Clostridium diff.	362-396
	Mycoplasma & Ureaplasma	323-343
	Pneumococcus	318-385
		(318-392)
Kali-i.	Chlamydia	379-384
	Clostridium diff.	362-396
	Cryptococcus	353-420
	Mycoplasma & Ureaplasma	323-420
		(323-420)
Kali-mur.	Termibacter	n.a.
	Pneumococcus	318-385

Table 6 (continued)

HOMEOPATHIC REMEDY	PATHOGEN	RESONANCE FREQUENCIES KHz†
Kali-s.	Aerobacter Pneumococcus	374 318-392 (318-392)
Kreosotum	Chlamydia Herpes vir. Mycobact. tub. Yersinia	379-384 291-420 430-434 184-378* (184-420)
Lachesis	Bac. Morgan Malaria Propionbact. acne Rickettsia	n.a. 372-442 383-389 128-361 (128-442)
Lobelia	Klebsiella	416-422
Lycopodium	Enterococcus	325*
Mag-mur.	Yersinia	184-378
Medorrinum	Neisseria gon.	334
Merc-corr.	Clostridium diff. E-coli EBV CMV Coxsackie vir. Hepatitis Meningococcus Mycobact. tub. Rotavirus Staphylococcus Streptococcus	362-396 356-392 372-381 408-411 360-366 418 n.a. 430-434 n.a. 376-381 318-385 (318-434)

Table 6 (continued)

HOMEOPATHIC REMEDY	PATHOGEN	RESONANCE FREQUENCIES KHz†
Merc-cy.	E-coli	356-392
	EBV	372-381
	CMV	408-411
	Coxsackie vir.	360-366
	Mycobact. tub.	430-434
	Rotavirus	n.a.
	Staphylococcus	376-381
	Streptococcus	318-385
		(318-434)
Merc-dul.	EBV	372-381
	CMV	408-411
	Coxsackie vir.	360-366
	Mycobact. tub.	430-434
	Rotavirus	n.a.
		(408-434)
Merc-i-fl.	EBV	372-381
	CMV	408-411
	Coxsackie vir.	360-366
	Mycobact. tub.	430-434
	Rotavirus	n.a.
		(408-434)
Merc-i-r.	EBV	372-381
	E-coli	365-392
	CMV	408-411
	Coxsackie vir.	360-366
	Meningococcus	n.a.
	Mycobact. tub.	430-434
	Rickettsia	128-361*
	Rotavirus	n.a.
	Staphylococcus	376-381
		(128-434)

Table 6 (continued)

HOMEOPATHIC REMEDY	PATHOGEN	RESONANCE FREQUENCIES KHz†
Merc-sol.	EBV	372-381
	E-coli	356-392
	CMV	408-411
	Coxsackie vir.	360-366
	Cryptococcus	353-420*
	Gardnerella	338-343
	Meningococcus	n.a.
	Mycobact. tub.	430-434
	Rickettsia	128-361*
	Rotavirus	n.a.
	Staphylococcus	376-381
	Streptococcus	318-385
		(128-434)
Merc-viv.	EBV	372-381
	E-coli	356-392
	Chlamydia	379-384
	CMV	408-411
	Coxsackie vir.	360-366
	Meningococcus	n.a.
	Mycobact. tub.	430-434
	Rotavirus	n.a.
	Staphylococcus	376-381
	Streptococcus	318-385
		(318-434)
Mezereum	Proteus	324-413
Nat-ars.	Enterococcus	325*
	EBV	372-381
	Pneumococcus	318-385
		(318-385)
Nat-mur.	Herpes vir.	291-420

Table 6 (continued)

HOMEOPATHIC REMEDY	PATHOGEN	RESONANCE FREQUENCIES KHz†
Nux-v.	Clostridium diff.	362-396
	Hepatitis vir.	414-421
	Malaria	372-442
		(362-442)
Petroleum	Hepatitis vir.	414-421
Phosphorus	Aspergillus	365-420*
	Campylobacter & Helicobacter	355-368
	Enterococcus	325*
	Mucor	288; 353-392*
	Mycoplasma & Ureaplasma	323-343
	Mycobact. tub.	430-434
	Streptococcus	318-385
	Proteus	324-413
		(288-434)
Phytolacca	Streptococcus	318-385
Podophylum	Bac. coli	n.a.
	Rotavirus	n.a.
Psorinum	Herpes vir.	291-420
Pulsatilla	Streptococcus	318-385
Pyrogen	Chlamidia	379-384
	Mycoplasma & Ureaplasma	323-343
	Proteus	324-413
		(323-413)
Rhus-tox.	CMV	408-411
	Herpes vir.	291-420
	Streptococcus	318-385
		(291-420)
Rumex	Chlamydia	379-384

Table 6 (continued)

HOMEOPATHIC REMEDY	PATHOGEN	RESONANCE FREQUENCIES KHz†
Sabina	Chlamydia Neiseria gon.	379-384 333-337 (333-384)
Sanicula	Chlamydia	379-384
Sarsaparilla	Enterococcus E-coli Gardnerella	325* 356-392 338-343 (325-392)
Scrophularia	Mycobact. tub.	430-434
Secale	Schistosoma/Bilharzia Trichinella sp.	353-473 403-406 (353-406)
Sepia	Herpes vir. Proteus	291-420 324-413 (291-420)
Spigelia	Enterobius	420-426
Spongia	Mycoplasma & Ureaplasma	323-343
Sticta	Mycoplasma & Ureaplasma Klebsiella Streptococcus	323-343 401-417 318-385 (318-417)
Strophantus	Herpes vir.	291-420
Sulphur	Hepatitis Herpes vir.	414-421 291-420 (291-421)
Sulph-i.	Clostridium diff.	362-396

Table 6 (continued)

HOMEOPATHIC REMEDY	PATHOGEN	RESONANCE FREQUENCIES KHz[†]
Tellurium	Herpes vir.	291-420
Terebinthina	Serratia	n.a.
Teucrium	CMV	408-411
Thuja	Herpes vir. Neisseria gon. Yersinia	291-420 333-337 184-378* (184-420)
Urtica urens	Streptococcus	318-385
Veratrum-album	Campylobacter & Helicobacter Rickettsia Salmonella Yersinia	355-368 128-361 329-355 184-378* (128-378)
Zinc-met.	Campylobacter & Helicobacter Schistosoma/Bilharzia	355-368 353-473 (353-473)
Zinc-phos.	Campylobacter & Helicobacter	355-368
Zinc-pic.	Schistosoma/Bilharzia Guiardia lamblia Toxoplasma	353-473 421-426 395 (395-426)
Zinc-valer.	Schistosoma/Bilharzia	353-473

These resonance frequencies we found by testing with lactose granules, charged with vibration frequencies produced by the machine Driver Resonator.
†*According to Clark, H. R. (1995).*

TABLE 7
SOME PARASITES AND HOMEOPATHIC REMEDIES CONFIRMED BY EAV TEST AS SPECIFIC FOR THESE PARASITES

PATHOGEN	HOMEOPATHIC REMEDY
Amoeba	Aloe*, Ac-acet., Ac-p., Bry., Carb-v. (and oxidants)
Ascaris	Cina*
Babesia	China, Cupr-met.
Bilharzia (Schistosoma)	Secale*, Ant-t., Zinc-met., Zinc-pic., Zinc-valer.
Echinococcus	Apis*, Hydrastis*
Enterobius verm.	Cina*, Carbo-an.*, Spig., Calc-c.
Guiardia lamblia	Berberis*, Zinc-picr.
Malaria	Bellis-per., Borax, China, Chin-ars., Chin-sulph.,Carb-v., Lach., Nux-v.
Taenia	Zinc-picr.
Trichinella sp.	Secale*
Trichomonas hom.	Helonias*, Clematis*
Toxoplasma gondii	Zinc-picr.*, Calc-c., Cina.

Note: For all of these pathogens, the herbal tincture Paragon works very well.

* *According to Usupov, G. A. (2000)*

REFERENCES

Adey, W. R. (1988) *The Cellular Microenvironment and Signaling through Cell Membranes.* Loma Linda, CA: Loma Linda University School of Medicine. pp. 81–106.

Akimov, A., & Tarasenko, V. (1992) Models of polarized states of the physical vacuum and torsion fields. *Soviet Physics Journal, 35* (March), 214.

Bleker, M. M. (1993) *Blood Examination in Darkfield, According to Prof. Dr. Gunther Enderlein.* Germany: Semmelweis-Verlag.

Bohm, D. (1987) *Wholeness and the Implicate Order.* London: Routledge and Kegan Paul.

Boiadjiev, M. M. (2000) *Systematic Approach in Homeopathic Theory and Practice.* Sofia, Bulgaria: Elena Kirkova Publ.

Broxmeyer, L. (2003) *AIDS: What the Discoverer of HIV Never Admitted.* Chula Vista, CA: New Century Press. ISBN 1890035297.

Clark, H. R. (1995) *The Cure for All Diseases.* San Diego: ProMotion Publishing.

Deacon, J. The University of Edinburgh, UK, Institute of Cell and Molecular Biology. http://helios.bto.ed.ac.uk/bto/microbes/proteus.htm

Delinik, A. (1991) A new medical model of the organism and its pathology. *The Berlin Journal on Research in Homeopathy, 1*(4/5), 243–253.

Delinik, A. (1999a) *Homeopathy, Scientifically Proved Facts and Possibilities.* Sofia: Association of Homeopathic Physicians in Bulgaria.

Delinik, A. (1999b) The wave-like behaviour between homeopathic remedies and the organism. *Homeopathia Internationalis Newsletter, 3.*

De Vernejoul, P., et al. (1985) Etude des meridiens d'acupuncture par les traceurs radioactifs. *Bulletin of the Academy of National Medicine, 169* (October), 1071–1075.

Diez-Gonzalez, F., Callaway, T. R., Kizoulis, M. G., & Russell, J. B. (1998) Grain feeding and dissemination of acid resistant Escherichia coli from cattle. *Science*, 281, 1666–1668.

Dumitrescu, I., & Kenyon, J. (1983) *Electrographic Imaging in Medicine and Biology.* Suffolk, UK: Neville Spearman.

Dupont, H. (1995) *Shigella Species.* In G. L. Mandele, J. E. Bennet, & R. Dolin, *Principles and Practice of Infectious Diseases (fourth edition),* New York: Churchill Livingstone, pp. 2033–2039.

Enderlein, G. (1916) Bacteria Cyclogeny. Prescott, AZ: Enderlein Enterprises. [Reprinted in German in 1981 by Semmelweis-Verlag]

Fredericks, G. (2001) *Darkfield Warriors.* Australia: New Look Biologics. p. 56.

Frost, F., Caun, G. F., & Calderon, R. L. (1998) *Emerging Infectious Diseases,* 4(4).

Gerber, R. (2001) *Vibrational Medicine (third edition).* Rochester, VT: Bear & Co.

Gottschall, E. (2003) *Breaking the Vicious Cycle (tenth edition).* Ontario: Kirkton Press.

Gracey, M. S. (1981) Nutrition, bacteria, and the gut. *British Medical Bulletin, 37,* 71–75.

Greene, B. (1999) *The Elegant Universe.* UK: Vintage.

Grigorova, N., & Djerekarova, V. (1996) Quantum photochemistry and homeopathy. *European Journal of Homoeopathy* (edited by G. Vitoulkas), 31–34.

Groves, C. (1998) *The John Hopkins Microbiology Newsletter, 17*(28).

Hahnemann, S. (1921) *Organon of Medicine (sixth edition).* Calcutta.

Harrison, E. (2003) *Masks of the Universe (second edition).* UK: Cambridge University Press.

Hawking, S. (1989) *A Brief History of Time.* UK: Bantam Books.

Herscu, P. (1996) *Stramonium, with an Introduction to Analysis Using Cycles and Segments.* Amherst, MA: New England School of Homoeopathy Press.

Ho, M. W., & Popp, F. A. (1989) *Gaia and the Evolution of Coherence.* Third Cameford Conference; Cornwall, UK; November 1989. http://www.i-sis.org.uk/gaia.php

Hunter, J. O. (1991) Food allergy or enterometabolic disorder? *Lancet, 338,* 495–496.

Jadin, C. L. (1999) *The Rickettsial and Para Rickettsial Approach of CFS and Related Disorders.* Johannesburg, South Africa.

Jadin, C. (2002) *A Disease Called Fatigue.* South Africa: HPH Publishing.

Johansen, E. (2003) *The South African Journal of Natural Medicine, 10,* 24.

Joung, S. H., Dobozin, B. S., & Miner, M. (1999) *Allergies, the Complete Guide to Diagnosis, Treatment, and Daily Management.* US: Penguin Putnam, a Plume Book.

Kent, J. (1996) *Repertory of the Homoeopathic Materia Medica.* New Delhi: B. Jain Publications.

Kenyon, J. N. (1992) *Modern Techniques of Acupuncture (volumes 1 and 2).* New York/UK: Thorsons.

Kiehn, R. M. (2002) *Integrable and Nonintegrable Structure in Shipov's Physical Vacuum.* University of Houston, Physics Dept. www.cartan. pair.com; rkiehn2352@aol.com

László, E. (2004) *Science and the Akashic Field.* Rochester, VT: Inner Traditions. pp. 27–35.

Lupitchev, L. N. (1992) *Electroacupuncture Diagnosis, Homeopathy and the Phenomenon of the Distance Action.* Moscow.

Luvsan, G. (1990) *Traditional and Modern Aspects of Eastern Reflexology (second edition)* [in Russian]. Moscow.

Mackie, T. J., & McCartney, J. E. (1978) *Medical Microbiology.* Churchill Livingstone. ISBN 0443017875.

Medzhitov, R., & Janeway, C. (2000) Innate immunity. *The New England Journal of Medicine, 343,* 338–344.

Murphy, R. (1996) *Homeopathic Medical Repertory.* Colorado: Hahnemann Academy of North America.

Mycology of Dermatophyte Infections. http://www.dermnetnz.org/fungal/mycology.html

Parikh, S. L., Venkatraman, G., DelGaudio, J. M. (2004) Invasive fungal sinusitis: A 15-year review from a single institution. Department of Otolaryngology – Head and Neck Surgery, Emory University School of Medicine. *American Journal of Rhinology, 18*(2) (March–April), 75–81.

Parker, C. A. (1968) *Photoluminescence of Solutions.* Amsterdam/London/New York: Elsevier.

Pert, C. (1997) *Molecules of Emotions.* US.

Playfair, J. (2004) *Living with Germs in Sickness and Health.* UK: Oxford University Press.

Poponin, V. *The DNA Phantom Effect: Direct Measurement of a New Field in the Vacuum Substructure.*

Popp, F. A. (2003) *Consciousness as Evolutionary Process Based on Coherent States.* www.lifescientists.de/publication/pub2003-04-11.htm

Popp, F. A., Gu, Q., Ho, M. W. (1994) In *Bioelectrodinamics and Biocommunication,* edited by K. Barhke. Singapore: World Scientific.

Pribram, K. (1982) *The Holographic Paradigm (and Other Paradoxes),* edited by Ken Wilber. Boulder, CO: Shambhala.

Pribram, K. (1984) The Holographic Hypothesis of Brain Function: A Meeting of Minds. In *Ancient Wisdom and Modern Science,* edited by S. Grof, Albany, NY: State University of New York Press.

Scott-Mumby, K. (1999) *Virtual Medicine.* Thorsons.

Shipov, G. I. (1998) *The Theory of the Physical Vacuum* [in Russian]. Moscow. ISBN 5727300118. [English edition published by the Russian Academy of Sciences]

Simeonova, N. K. (1989) *Homeopathy and Astrochemistry.* Kiev: Nord Kavkaz. [In Russian]

Stolberg, L., Rolfe, R., Gitlin, N., Merritt, J., Mam, L., Linderer, J. R., & Finegold, S. (1982) D-lactic acidosis due to abnormal flora. *The New England Journal of Medicine, 306,* 1344–1348.

Tanev P., & Vlahov A. (1995) *Principles of Bioresonance Diagnosis.* Tarnovo, Bulgaria: Plam Co. [In Bulgarian]

Tannock, G. W. (1995) *Normal Microflora.* Chapman & Hall.

Thurn, J. R., Pierpont, G. L., Ludvigsen, C. W., & Eckfeldt, H. (1985) D-lactate encephalopathy. *The American Journal of Medicine, 79,* 717–721.

Trowbridge, J. P., & Walker, M. (1986) *The Yeast Syndrome.* Bantam Books.

Usupov, G. A. (2000) *Energy–Information Medicine. Homeopathy, Homotoxicology, Electropuncture by Voll.* Moscow: Moskovskie Novosti Publications.

Vithoulkas, G. (1980) *The Science of Homeopathy.* New Delhi: B. Jain.

Voll, R. (1976) *Topographische lade der Electroakupunktur.* Uelzen: Medizinich Literaturische Verlagsgesellschalf MBH.

Voll, R. (1980) The phenomenon of medicine testing in acupuncture according to Voll. *American Acupuncture, 8,* 97–104.

Whitmont, Edward C. (1993) *The Alchemy of Healing.* Berkeley, CA: North Atlantic Books. p. 96.

Zinger, S. (2003) *The Good Gut Guide.* UK: Thorsons. p. 162.

INDEX

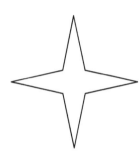
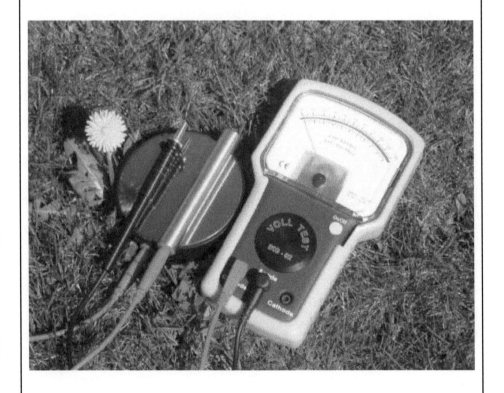

Lightning Source UK Ltd.
Milton Keynes UK
UKHW021250140222
398664UK00007B/1420